eHealth Solutions for Healthcare Disparities

eHealth Solutions for Healthcare Disparities

Edited by

Michael Christopher Gibbons, MD, MPH

Associate Director, Johns Hopkins Urban Health Institute (UHI)
Director, Center for Community HEALTH (CCH)
Assistant Professor of Public Health and Medicine,
Johns Hopkins Medical Institutions
Baltimore, Maryland

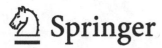 Springer

Michael Christopher Gibbons
Johns Hopkins Urban Health Institute
Baltimore, MD 21205
USA

ISBN 978-1-4419-2497-1   e-ISBN 978-0-387-72815-5

Printed on acid-free paper.

9 8 7 6 5 4 3 2 1

springer.com

Preface

Over the past decade a rapidly expanding body of literature has demonstrated the existence of healthcare disparities. While consensus has not emerged regarding the causes of disparities, they are generally thought to be related to provider, patient, and healthcare system factors. On the one hand, the current US healthcare system is oriented toward individualized acute care. Yet healthcare disparities by definition are a population level phenomenon. Individuals do not have disparities, groups and populations do. Thus population level data alone will not enable us to develop individualized interventions. Similarly, biologic, cellular, or molecular level data that is not informed by sociocultural realities has limited ability to help us craft the most appropriate interventions to address healthcare disparities. Rather knowledge from each of these levels of analysis must be sought, integrated, and evaluated. In so doing we will gain a far more relevant and informed understanding of healthcare disparities and have a better foundation from which to build clinical and behavioral interventions.

To develop the best interventions, several authorities have suggested the need for greater information technology research and investments. eHealth researchers may be able to make significant contributions in this area through research and its applications. Not surprisingly though, most individuals concerned about healthcare disparities have little knowledge of the fields of health information technologies or eHealth. Similarly, many working in the technology fields have only a cursory understanding of healthcare disparities. As such, the intent of this book is to draw together two unlikely bedfellows; the information technology fields and the sociobehavioral and population sciences, and to challenge readers to consider new possibilities and opportunities across the two disciplines.

In order to successfully accomplish this task the first section of this book contains several chapters discussing the field of healthcare disparities and current consensus on factors considered important in their causation. Because any serious consideration of computer technologies is not complete without a discussion of the role of the Internet, the second section of the book contains several chapters discussing the role of the Internet in society and emerging disparities in access and utilization of this technology. The third section of this book focuses on three computer- and technology-based themes most relevant to healthcare disparities, namely eHealth,

Medical Informatics, and Public Health Informatics. Finally, the last section of this book has several chapters pulling it all together. These chapters discuss future innovations in research that will be needed to foster a more informed and comprehensive understanding of healthcare disparities as well as policy opportunities for moving forward. The book ends with a chapter suggesting several ways in which technology may help us achieve the goal of reducing and eliminating healthcare disparities, some perhaps not previously considered. It is our hope that you find this book not only interesting, but also intellectually provocative to the point that you challenge old notions and conventions related to healthcare disparities and develop new technology-based collaborations to make the promise and the potential of technology strategies to address healthcare disparities, a reality.

M. Chris Gibbons
Editor

Contents

Section IV

Contributors

Michael Christopher Gibbons, MD, MPH, Associate Director, Johns Hopkins Urban Health Institute (UHI); Director, Center for Community HEALTH (CCH); Assistant Professor of Public Health and Medicine, Johns Hopkins Medical Institutions, Baltimore, MD

Anthony J Alberg, PhD, Johns Hopkins Bloomberg School of Public Health, Johns Hopkins Oncology Center, Baltimore, MD

David Ahern, PhD, National Program Director, Health e-Technologies Initiative, Brigham and Women's Hospital; Assistant Professor of Psychology (Psychiatry), Harvard Medical School, Boston, MA

Stephen Baylin, MD, Johns Hopkins School of Medicine, Johns Hopkins Oncology Center, Baltimore, MD

Malcolm Brock, MD, Johns Hopkins School of Medicine, Johns Hopkins Oncology Center, Baltimore, MD

Stephanie Chang, MD, MPH, Department of Medicine, Johns Hopkins School of Medicine, Baltimore, MD

Charles B. Eaton, MD, MS, Professor of Family Medicine, The Warren Alpert Medical School of Brown University; Director, Center for Primary Care and Prevention, Memorial Hospital of Rhode Island, Pawtucket, RI

Patricia Flatley Brennan, RN, PhD, FAAN, Moehlman Bascom Professor, School of Nursing and College of Engineering, University of Wisconsin-Madison, Madison, WI

C. Earl Fox, MD, MPH, Johns Hopkins Urban Health Institute, Johns Hopkins Bloomberg School of Public Health, Baltimore, MD

Thomas Glass, PhD, Johns Hopkins Bloomberg School of Public Health, Johns Hopkins Bloomberg School of Public Health Center on Aging and Health, Baltimore, MD

Bradford W. Hesse, PhD, National Cancer Institute, Bethesda, MD

Thomas A LaVeist, PhD, Johns Hopkins Bloomberg School of Public Health, Johns Hopkins Center for Health Disparities Solutions, Baltimore, MD

David Levine, MD, MPH, ScD, Johns Hopkins School of Medicine, Johns Hopkins Bloomberg School of Public Health, Baltimore, MD

Ruth Perot, MAT, Executive Director, Summit Health Institute for Research and Education, Washington, DC

Judith M. Phalen, MPH, Deputy Director, Health e-Technologies Initiative, Brigham and Women's Hospital, Boston, MA

Nadra Tyus, PhD, Post Doctoral Fellow, Johns Hopkins Urban Health Institute, Baltimore, MD

Rupa S Valdez, PhD.(candidate), Predoctoral Fellow, College of Engineering, University of Wisconsin-Madison, Madison, WI

Section I

1
An Overview of Healthcare Disparities

Michael Christopher Gibbons

Recognition of a Problem

By the early 1980s, Wennberg et al., using small area analysis and geographic information systems analytic techniques, demonstrated that a significant amount of nonrandom medical practice variability existed between clinical practices in different geographic locales, despite treating clinically similar patients (Barnes, O'Brien, Comstock, D'Arpa, & Donahue, 1985; McPherson, Wennberg, Hovind, & Clifford, 1982). In their study they examined the incidence of several common surgical procedures in seven hospital service areas in southern Norway, 21 sites in the United Kingdom, and 18 sites in the northeastern US. Although overall surgical rates were higher in the US than in the United Kingdom or Norway, there was significant variability in surgical rates among sites. In addition the variability was similar across all the three countries. In fact there was surprising consistency among countries in the rank order of variability for most procedures: tonsillectomy, hemorrhoidectomy, hysterectomy, and prostatectomy varied more from area to area than did appendectomy, hernia repair, or cholecystectomy. Thus this variation appeared to be nonrandom and not related to the organization or financing of care across the three countries (McPherson et al.).

A large analysis by Barnes seemed to corroborate Weinberg's findings of differential healthcare delivery in relation to geography. In this study Barnes et al. examined over 140,000 surgical procedures performed in Massachusetts in 1980. The location of the facilities where these procedures occurred was mapped and subdivided into more than 150 geographically defined areas across the state. The resulting analysis revealed that per capita surgical rates across geographic areas were significantly (two-to threefold) different and seemingly unrelated to clinical characteristics of patients served. Some surgical procedures were even being provided at rates substantially different from the statewide rate (Barnes et al., 1985).

By the early 1990s the evidence of disparate care provision in the US healthcare system continued to mount with the emergence of data from the Harvard Medical Practice Study (Brennan, Leape, Laird, Localio, & Hiatt, 1990; Brennan, Leape, et al., 1991; Leape et al., 1991). This study was undertaken, in part, to evaluate risk factors related to injury caused by the healthcare system. This comprehensive study was

3

based on more than 30,000 medical records from 51 randomly chosen hospitals in New York (Brennan, Hebert, et al., 1991), and revealed that a significant amount of injury to patients from medical practice occurred in this sample of the healthcare system. It also found that these adverse events were not randomly distributed with many injuries being the result of substandard care (Brennan, Leape, et al., 1991; Brennan et al., 1990; Leape et al.). An examination of hospital characteristics associated with these adverse events revealed that in addition to other factors, a significantly higher risk of adverse events was found among hospitals serving large proportions of minority patients. In fact in multivariate analysis, the only factor that remained significantly associated with an increased risk of adverse events due to negligence was treatment of a large proportion of minority patients (Brennan, Hebert, et al.). Although the authors could not explain the cause of these findings they suggested that they reflected the quality of care delivered in hospitals, not patient behavioral factors or other clinical factors related to the natural history of patient disease (Brennan, Hebert, et al.).

Thus by the late 1990s, growing evidence suggested that issues of racial and ethnic healthcare differences, practice variation, and substandard care, may all be related to the quality of health care experienced by patients. About this time Fiscella published his paper entitled "Inequality in Quality," in which he called attention to issues of healthcare quality and healthcare disparities as related issues of healthcare organizational capacity. He further contended that national efforts to eliminate racial and ethnic disparities in health care and national healthcare quality improvement initiatives represented two inseparable components of providing high-quality health care for all citizens (Fiscella, Franks, Gold, & Clancy, 2000). Thus for the first time in the US, it was suggested that health care should not be considered high quality as long as significant quality gaps and healthcare disparities remained.

Synthesizing the Scientific Evidence on Healthcare Disparities

To help bring clarity to these issues, the Institute of Medicine released the first of several reports highlighting and summarizing the scientific evidence concerning issues of differential health status, culture, behavior, communication, substandard care/medical errors, and healthcare quality (Haynes & Smedley, 1999; Institute of Medicine, 2001, 2002, 2003; IOM Committee on Quality of Healthcare in America, 2001; Kohn, Corrigan, & Donaldson, 2000; Smedley, Stith, & Nelson, 2003). The first report entitled "To Err is Human; Building a safer healthcare system" helped quantify the magnitude of the quality problem in the eyes of the public. This report suggested that the number of people who die each year from medical errors may be as high as 98,000 (Kohn et al.). With this assertion, no longer could poor outcomes or healthcare quality issues be seen as limited to the poor, to those patients who make poor health decisions or to the uninsured. This report suggested that providers and the healthcare system themselves played a role in the ultimate healthcare outcomes of patients.

Two reports followed that were released the following year in 2001. The first entitled "Envisioning the National Health Care Quality Report" (Institute of Medicine, 2001) laid the groundwork for a National Healthcare Quality Report. This would be national systematic annual evaluation of healthcare quality in the US. The second entitled "Crossing the quality chasm: A new health system for the 21st century" (IOM Committee on Quality of Healthcare in America, 2001) advocated a new vision for the future of health care. This vision was based not only on the growing realization of the existence of significant health quality gaps in the US healthcare system, but also on the notion that working harder within the context of the then current system, would not likely yield significant improvement. Rather, fundamental changes in the healthcare system would be needed (IOM Committee on Quality of Healthcare in America). The authors argued that although science and medical technology had advanced rapidly in recent years, the healthcare system in its then current capacity was lagging in its ability to communicate effectively with patients and to adequately coordinate care among patients suffering from chronic diseases who are in need of nonhospital-based care (IOM Committee on Quality of Healthcare in America). In the view of this committee, health care in the future should be of high quality in each of six critical dimensions. These include (1) Safety – providing health care that does not cause patient injuries, (2) Effective – providing evidence-based healthcare services to all who need them at the needed level/amount, (3) Patient centered – providing health care that is responsive to individual patient preferences, needs, and values, (4) Timely – providing health care without harmful delays, (5) Efficient – providing health care in a way that minimizes waste of resources, and (6) Equitable – providing health care of a consistent quality to all patients at all times, in any location or setting. Although it was not explicitly stated, this committee appeared to feel strongly that a healthcare system that achieved these goals among all patients would be a system that would also have successfully addressed healthcare disparities among racial and ethnic minorities.

Unfortunately, achieving these goals would not come easily. The growing diversity of the US population along with the quality problems in the US healthcare system strongly suggested that prevailing notions of health communication, patient behavior, and patient–provider interaction needed to be reexamined, particularly among minority populations. There was a growing realization that the recent advances in diagnostic testing and medical treatment along with quantum leaps in our understanding of disease at the cellular, molecular, and genetic levels were not sufficient to guarantee optimal health. The widespread documentation of healthcare disparities suggested that psychological factors, human behaviors, social ties as well as family and community life might also be important determinants of healthcare outcomes which should be considered more closely and integrated better into the context of US health care (Singer & Ryff, 2001). In short, the social and behavioral sciences which traditionally had not been considered within the domain of health care were perhaps linked to illness, health, and healthcare outcomes (Singer & Ryff).

This represented new ground for US health care. As such the IOM commissioned a report entitled "Speaking of health: Assessing health communication strategies for diverse populations." This study explored the dynamics and challenges of effective cross-cultural communication. It examined the need for more science-based communication interventions, and the role of socio-cultural factors on patient beliefs and behaviors in health care (Institute of Medicine, 2002). While the committee was unable to determine, from the then existing literature, if socioculturally determined knowledge could improve healthcare communications or enhance efforts to address health disparities, they were able to recommend that (1) underserved individuals and communities should be encouraged to participate actively in the construction of health com-munication campaigns in their communities, (2) practitioners should employ evidence-based, multicomponent programs that integrate communication with access to services, and (3) novel technology-based communication strategies to improve the health of diverse populations should be explored (Institute of Medicine, 2002).

Because, as the report highlighted, the precise nature and impact of the associa-tion between the sociobehavioral sciences and the medicoclinical sciences could not be definitively characterized, medical research conducted and supported via the National Institutes of Health should begin to focus on elucidating this knowl-edge in addition to understanding the biology of disease. To this end, the director of the Office of Behavioral and Social Science Research at the National Institutes of Health requested assistance from the National Research Council (NRC) to develop a research plan to guide the NIH in supporting an integrative approach to health research (Singer & Ryff, 2001). The report entitled "New Horizons in Health; An Integrative Approach" articulated ten priority areas for research investment that would integrate the behavioral, social, and biomedical sciences into healthcare research. In their report the NRC recommended a focus on predis-ease pathways or the identification of early and long-term biological, behavioral, psychological, and social precursors to disease. It was also recommended that a focus on the identification of biological, behavioral, psychological, and social factors that contribute to health and resilience, not just disease, morbidity and mortality would likely yield insights not possible using a deficit model of health. It was recommended that there should be an emphasis on environmentally induced gene expression. Such a focus carried the promise of significantly enhancing our understanding of the links between recently derived molecular genetic processes and biological, behavioral, psychological, and social realities. Finally, the NRC recommended a distinct focus on the impact of aggregate neigh-borhood, community-level, and larger population-level factors on health and healthcare outcomes.

Due to the significant scope of each of these recommendations, there existed the potential to lose focus on the healthcare disparities issue. Thus the NRC recommended that a specific focus on inequalities in health and specifically on interventions to address these inequalities be maintained in healthcare research. Also, because many of these recommendations represented fairly radical departures from the status quo in health care and biomedical research, the NRC recommended a focus on new multilevel, integrative evaluative methodologies, and study designs as well as a focus on the development of a new type of clinical researcher, one who possesses the necessary skills and aptitude to conduct this type of integrative and transdisciplinary work (Singer & Ryff, 2001).

The culmination of work on quality and healthcare disparities came with the 2003 release of a report entitled "Unequal Treatment: Confronting Racial and Ethnic Disparities in Health Care" (Smedley et al., 2003). In this report, the IOM Committee on Understanding and Eliminating Racial and Ethnic Disparities in Health Care was specifically charged with assessing the extent and potential sources of racial and ethnic disparities in health care that are not otherwise attributable to access to care, ability to pay, or insurance coverage. The committee was also to provide recommendations regarding potential interventions to eliminate these healthcare disparities (Smedley et al.). The committee found evidence that, within the US, even among the middle class and individuals with access to health care, racial and ethnic disparities indeed existed. In some cases these disparities were increasing and were likely related to patient factors, provider factors, socio-economic factors, and broader factors related to historic and contemporary race-based bias (Smedley et al.). These disparities were, with few exceptions, remarkably consistent across a wide range of illnesses and healthcare services including cardiovascular disease, cancer, end stage renal disease, diabetes care, kidney transplantation, pediatric care, maternal and child health, mental health, rehabilitative and nursing home services, and many surgical services (Smedley et al.). In a few cases the committee found that minorities were actually more likely than Whites to experience certain procedures (bilateral orchiectomy, leg amputations) and that there was little evidence that these disparities were the result of patient preferences (Smedley et al.).

Time Trends and Recent Data

Even before the release of the IOM reports, the US congress became involved by passing the Healthcare Research and Quality Act of 1999 which directed the Agency for Healthcare Research and Quality (AHRQ) to develop an annual National Healthcare Quality Report and an Annual National Healthcare Disparities Report. Building on the IOM's Quality Chasm report which outlined six dimensions of high-quality health care, AHRQ developed a disparities conceptual framework that incorporated these quality dimensions with special emphasis on the equity domain (Agency for Healthcare Research and Quality, 2003).

To date, four annual reports have been released, with the first becoming available in 2004. The initial report provided the baseline information needed for prospective evaluation of progress toward reducing healthcare disparities and for the first time measured the magnitude of these disparities from a national perspective (Agency for Healthcare Research and Quality, 2003). The major findings and conclusions of this first report include the demonstration that racial and ethnic healthcare disparities are a pervasive national problem affecting all parts of the healthcare continuum, across all diseases and medical conditions (Agency for Healthcare Research and

Quality, 2003). The report also found that healthcare disparities were associated with poorly managed care, avoidable complications, significant morbidity, disability, access to care barriers, and excessive personal and societal costs (Agency for Healthcare Research and Quality, 2003). The second report, released in 2004 largely echoed these findings, but also suggested that some areas appeared to have been improving including late stage breast cancer diagnoses and childhood immunization rates between Whites and African-Americans (Agency for Healthcare Research and Quality, 2004). In contrast, the 2005 report found that many of the gains outlined in the 2004 report were no longer improving while others were in fact getting worse. It also showed that low income individuals regardless of race or ethnicity often experienced the largest disparities in healthcare quality (Agency for Healthcare Research and Quality, 2005). Finally this report also suggested a need for a shift in national focus from merely documenting disparities to finding ways to reduce or eliminate the gaps (Agency for Healthcare Research and Quality, 2005). Not surprisingly the 2006 report also documented inconsistent improvements and some worsening in US healthcare disparities (Agency for Healthcare Research and Quality, 2006).

Summary

Over the last two decades research from several distinct lines of investigation have coalesced to underscore the relationship between medical care, biophysiologic processes, sociocultural, and other environmental influences on healthcare outcomes generally and healthcare disparities specifically. In the early 1980s researchers examining variability in clinical practice patterns found nonrandom distributions in care across geographic locations. In the mid 1980s the report of the Secretary's Task Forces on Black and Minority Health (Department of Health and Human Services, 1985) highlighted the fact that the health of Blacks and minorities significantly lagged behind that of Whites in the US. By the early 1990s large scale epidemiologic studies confirmed earlier findings of nonrandom distribution of clinical practice patterns and the association between substandard care and low income and minority patients. These early findings encouraged a focus on healthcare quality problems within the US healthcare system. Upon closer examination it was revealed that problems associated with quality and healthcare disparities were in fact linked and should be considered together. In the case of healthcare disparities, the recent clinical and technological advances that had been achieved appeared insufficient to guarantee the reduction of healthcare disparities. As such, efforts were undertaken to better clarify the impact of "nonmedical" communications and social factors on healthcare outcomes. These investigations highlighted the need to better integrate the biomedical and sociobehavioral disciplines in current health care and clinical practice to improve quality and address disparities among an increasingly diverse population. In addition, national efforts to document and quantify both the magnitude of the healthcare disparities and healthcare quality problems were needed. These evaluations documented the pervasiveness of healthcare disparities at all levels of health care. They also suggested that close to 100,000 people may die each year from healthcare quality related issues and medical errors. This spurred a significant amount of planning to develop interventions and monitor progress at the national level. To date, much has been accomplished to improve overall healthcare quality and healthcare disparities. While some quality indicators and healthcare disparities have improved several others have not and some even worsened. As such, while progress is occurring, more work needs to be done.

References

Agency for Healthcare Research and Quality. (2003). *The national healthcare disparities report*. Washington, DC: Author.

Agency for Healthcare Research and Quality. (2004). *The national healthcare disparities report*. Washington, DC: Author.

Agency for Healthcare Research and Quality. (2005). *The national healthcare disparities report*. Washington, DC: Author.

Agency for Healthcare Research and Quality. (2006). *The national healthcare disparities report*. Washington, DC: Author.

Barnes, B. A., O'Brien, E., Comstock, C., D'Arpa, D. G., & Donahue, C. L. (1985). Report on variation in rates of utilization of surgical services in the Commonwealth of Massachusetts. *JAMA: The Journal of the American Medical Association, 254*, 371–375.

Brennan, T. A., Hebert, L. E., Laird, N. M., Lawthers, A., Thorpe, K. E., Leape, L. L., et al. (1991). Hospital characteristics associated with adverse events and substandard care. *JAMA: The Journal of the American Medical Association, 265*, 3265–3269.

Brennan, T. A., Leape, L. L., Laird, N. M., Hebert, L., Localio, A. R., Lawthers, A. G., et al. (1991). Incidence of adverse events and negligence in hospitalized patients. Results of the Harvard Medical Practice Study I. *The New England Journal of Medicine, 324*, 370–376.

Brennan, T. A., Leape, L. L., Laird, N. M., Localio, A. R., & Hiatt, H. H. (1990). Incidence of adverse events and negligent care in hospitalized patients. *Transactions of the Association of American Physicians, 103*, 137–144.

Department of Health and Human Services. (1985). *Report of the secretary's task forces on black and minority health*. Washington, DC: Author.

Fiscella, K., Franks, P., Gold, M. R., & Clancy, C. M. (2000). Inequality in quality: Addressing socioeconomic, racial, and ethnic disparities in health care. *JAMA: The Journal of the American Medical Association, 283*, 2579–2584.

Haynes, M., & Smedley, B. D. (1999). *The unequal burden of cancer*. Washington, DC: National Academy Press.

Institute of Medicine. (2001). *Envisioning the national healthcare quality report*. Washington, DC: National Academy Press.

Institute of Medicine. (2002). *Speaking of health: Assessing health communication strategies for diverse populations*. Washington, DC: National Academy Press.

Institute of Medicine. (2003). *Priority areas for national action: Transforming healthcare quality*. Washington, DC: National Academy Press.

IOM Committee on Quality of Healthcare in America. (2001). *Crossing the quality chasm: A new health system for the 21st century*. Washington, DC: National Academy Press.

Kohn, L., Corrigan, J., & Donaldson, M. (2000). *Too err is human: Building a safer health system*. Washington, DC: National Academy Press.

Leape, L. L., Brennan, T. A., Laird, N., Lawthers, A. G., Localio, A. R., Barnes, B. A., et al. (1991). The nature of adverse events in hospitalized patients. Results of the Harvard Medical Practice Study II. *The New England Journal of Medicine, 324*, 377–384.

McPherson, K., Wennberg, J. E., Hovind, O. B., & Clifford, P. (1982). Small-area variations in the use of common surgical procedures: An international comparison of New England, England, and Norway. *The New England Journal of Medicine, 307*, 1310–1314.

Singer, B. H., & Ryff, C. D. (2001). *New horizons in health: An integrative approach*. Washington, DC: National Academy Press.

Smedley, B. D., Stith, A. Y., & Nelson, A. R. (2003). *Unequal treatment: Confronting racial and ethnic disparities in healthcare*. Washington, DC: National Academy Press.

2
Provider Factors in Healthcare Disparities

Michael Christopher Gibbons

Several factors related to healthcare providers may be associated with healthcare disparities. Communication is fundamental to the healthcare process. Patient–provider communication is a multidimensional concept relating in part to both providers and patients. This chapter will discuss those aspects of patient–provider communication more closely related to the provider. Chapter 3 will discuss those patient–provider communication issues more closely related to patients.

Provider Communication

Most of the research being conducted prior to 1990 on the relationship between communication and healthcare outcomes came from European (British, Dutch, and American) studies with relatively little work conducted on other populations. In addition, the medical and communication models originating with these ethnic traditions considered the ideal doctor–patient relationship as somewhat paternalistic with the patients receiving and obeying medical instructions (Ong, de Haes, Hoos, & Lammes, 1995; Roter & Hall, 1993). Early investigators studied the technical or medical competency aspects of the doctor–patient visit, the degree to which the physicians responded to nonsomatic or psychosomatic issues and the degree to which open, secure, and workable relationships were established (Roter & Hall).

The motives underlying physician communication have also been studied. Provider motives have been defined as instrumental or socioemotional. Instrumental communication is communication that is focused on the so-called "cure" aspects of treatment (i.e., signs, symptoms, tests, treatments, side effects). Socioemotional communication is that communication that is focused on the so-called "care"-oriented behaviors (i.e., feelings, emotions, daily functioning, coping) (Ong et al., 1995). Most of the communications and health quality literature have focused on instrumental communication and particularly the information giving and seeking behaviors of doctors. These studies suggest that the amount of information given during the medical visit appears to increase as patient expressions of questioning and concern increase (Ong et al.). Also, increased physician-affective behaviors, including listening without interruption and use of first names, are associated with improved patient–provider communication.

Both verbal and nonverbal communications have been investigated in relation to healthcare outcomes. Nonverbal communication refers to tone of voice, eye contact, facial expressions, touch, and physical distance. Unfortunately, no single systematic approach has been used to codify these interactions and thus conclusions derived from this literature are difficult (Ong et al., 1995).

The study of the physician's vocabulary in the medical encounter is an area of active research. One study by Hadlow and Pitts demonstrated that common medical terms used by physicians and medical professionals are often misunderstood by patients (Roter & Hall, 1993). More recently a national survey conducted by the Commonwealth Fund found that problematic communication between physicians and patients occurred more often among English-speaking African-Americans, Hispanics, and Asian-Americans than Whites (Collins et al., 2002). These problems are heightened among patients who do not speak English as their primary language. This study also found that compared to White patients, African-Americans, Hispanics, and Asian-Americans were less likely to have great confidence in their doctors, less likely to be as involved in their own care as they would like and less likely to have as much time with their doctors as they would like (Collins et al.). Unfortunately, these problems are not unique to minority populations. This same study found that approximately 18% of all adults with healthcare visits in the recent past reported problems communicating with their doctors (Collins et al.).

Provider Communication and Select Healthcare Outcomes

Studies investigating the influence of language and communication on patient outcomes have largely been focused on three major areas – satisfaction, compliance, and physiologic outcomes. While the vast majority of the work has been in the satisfaction and compliance areas, each category will be briefly discussed below.

Patient Satisfaction

Many studies have been done investigating the relationship between information seeking or provision by a physician and patient satisfaction (Williams, Weinman, & Dale, 1998). Most, but not all, studies of physician information sharing found that provision of information by doctors to patients is associated with increases in patient satisfaction. In contrast though, a physician's spending increased amounts of time on a patient's history was associated with decreases in patient satisfaction (Williams et al.).

Studies have also been conducted evaluating the link between patient satisfaction and the nature of the doctor–patient relationship. The personal manner (bedside manner) has been associated with patient satisfaction. Physicians displaying behaviors such as being friendly, approving, engaging in social nonmedical conversation with patients, those who use encouraging, empathetic behaviors, and those physicians who engage in partnership building during the consultation are physicians who tend to have higher satisfaction rates among their patients (Roter & Hall, 1993; Roter, Hall, & Katz, 1987). It is unclear if physician's tone of voice or physician's affect significantly impacts patient satisfaction. Among the studies investigating this idea, the results are mixed with some studies finding a positive association and others finding a negative association with patient satisfaction (Roter & Hall; Roter et al.).

Finally, communication style and its relationship to patient satisfaction have been evaluated. In general, a disease-focused approach is perceived by patients as being doctor-led and an approach in which the doctor is focusing on his own agenda. On the other hand, a patient-centered approach is perceived by patients as being patient led and one where the doctor is listening and responding to the concerns of the patient. Many studies in this area find that higher rates of patient satisfaction are associated with higher degrees of patient-centered communication.

Patient Compliance

Early studies of patient compliance were only able to demonstrate weak associations between enhanced communication and patient compliance (Roter, 1989). More recently it has been suggested that patients with language barriers may be *less* likely to receive a follow-up appointment, but if given one, patients with language barriers are equally likely to keep a follow-up appointment as those without language barriers (Sarver & Baker, 2000).

The term "adherence" is increasingly used to reflect the patient perspective. Adherence is defined as a collaborative effect of healthcare providers and consumers to achieve mutually agreed health goals (Rose, Kim, Dennison, & Hill, 2000). It is estimated that only 50% of patients in the general population are adherent to long-term medical regimens (Charles, Good, Hanusa, Chang, & Whittle, 2003).

Although studies directly investigating adherence across racial and ethnic groups are few, some studies suggest that African-Americans and other special populations may have lower rates of adherence (Charles et al., 2003) as compared to Whites. On the other hand, increased adherence is associated with patient satisfaction and increased physician-affective behaviors (Hill et al., 1999; Rose et al., 2000).

Physiologic Outcomes and Healthcare Utilization

Few studies evaluating the association between communication and physiologic outcomes have been done. Yet, the available evidence suggests that less physician-controlling behavior during the visit, more expressions of affect, and more information given by the physician are associated with improvements in blood pressure, glucose control, and functional status (Kaplan, Greenfield, & Ware, 1989; Orth, Stiles, Scherwitz, Hennrikus, & Vallbona, 1987). Additionally, a few studies have linked enhanced physician communication with improvements in recovery from surgery, decreased utilization of pain medicines, and decreased length of stay in hospital (Mumford, Schlesinger, & Glass, 1982; Roter & Hall, 1993).

Provider Communication and Healthcare Disparities

It has been hypothesized that communication-related factors may contribute to healthcare disparities in potentially three ways. They are (1) disparate care may be provided by doctors in the context of total ignorance, (2) disparate care might be appropriate given the medical nature of populations of patients, and (3) doctors might be affected by the same biases and stereotypes that affect others in the population (Roter & Hall, 1993). Admittedly though, there is no consensus on these issues and the relative importance of these factors is hotly debated (Smedley, Stith, & Nelson, 2003).

A study by Cooper-Patrick et al. suggests that African-American patients experience shorter, more physician-dominated, less patient-centered visits than White patients (Smedley et al., 2003). As previously stated, other studies investigating the role of race/ethnicity and communication have largely been done in Eurocentric groups (Smedley et al.). While these studies do not include minorities of African, Caribbean, or North American descent, they still generally demonstrate health-related differences between European subgroup social classes (Roter & Hall, 1993; Smedley et al.). Negative stereotypes, bias, and prejudices of disadvantaged populations may affect the way doctors interact with individuals from those population groups (Smedley et al.).

Bias and Discrimination Among Healthcare Providers

Several studies suggest that while physicians, like other members of society, may find prejudice unacceptable and contradictory to personal and professional values, providers may not always recognize prejudice in their own behavior (Smedley et al., 2003). As outlined in Chap. 1, the Harvard Medical Practice Study (Brennan, Leape, et al., 1991; Brennan, Leape, Laird, Localio, & Hiatt, 1990; Leape et al.,

1991) was based on more than 30,000 medical records from 51 randomly chosen hospitals in New York (Brennan, Hebert, et al., 1991). This study revealed that a significant amount of injury to patients from medical practice occurred in this sample of healthcare system. It also found that these adverse events were not randomly distributed in the sample and that many injuries were the result of substandard care (Brennan, Leape, et al., 1991; Brennan et al., 1990; Leape et al.). In addition, a significantly higher risk of adverse events was found among hospitals serving large proportions of minority patients. In fact, in multivariate analysis, the only factor that remained significantly associated with an increased risk of adverse events due to negligence was the treatment of a large proportion of minority patients (Brennan, Hebert, et al.). Although the authors could not explain the cause of these findings, they suggested that the findings of the study and, in particular, the findings related to adverse events due to negligence reflected the quality of care delivered by doctors to patients, and not patient-behavioral factors or other clinical factors related to the natural history of patient's disease (Brennan, Hebert, et al.).

More recently, in a highly publicized study, Schulman studied physician recommendations for the management of chest pain (Schulman et al., 1999). In this study, physicians were shown video vignettes of patients who were actually trained actors portraying the same symptoms of coronary artery disease. The patients varied only by race (Whites vs. Black), sex, age (55 vs. 70), coronary risk, and results of an exercise test. Schulman found that physicians were less likely to recommend cardiac catheterization for women and African-Americans (Schulman et al.). While the magnitude of the findings and the statistical tests used in the analyses has been criticized, the existence of a difference is generally accepted. In two related studies, LaViest demonstrated that White cardiac patients are more likely to receive a special referral for coronary angiography (LaVeist, Arthur, Morgan, Plantholt, & Rubinstein, 2003) or cardiac rehabilitation (Gregory, LaVeist, & Simpson, 2006) than similar African-American cardiac patients.

Several studies suggest that physicians prescribe pain medications differentially among White and minority patients. Among patients discharged from an urban ER, Knox et al. demonstrated that Hispanics and Whites were less likely to be prescribed certain pain medicines than similar White patients (LaVeist, 2002). Similar findings have been documented among cancer patients (Bernabei et al., 1998; Cleeland, Gonin, Baez, Loehrer, & Pandya, 1997). A study by Morrison et al. suggests that the problem with prescription pain medications may go beyond that of the physician. In this study of New York City pharmacies, Morrison found that of 347 pharmacies, 51% did not have adequate supplies of certain pain medicines needed for patients with severe pain (Morrison, Wallenstein, Natale, Senzel, & Huang, 2000). In addition, those pharmacies with inadequate drug supplies were more likely to be in predominately non-White neighborhoods. According to the interviews with the pharmacists involved in this study, fear of theft, low demand, additional paperwork demand, regulatory oversight, and monitoring of these medicines were the major reasons for the inadequate supply of pain medicines (Morrison et al.). In sum then, these studies appear to indicate that racial and ethnic disparities in health care are related to differential patterns of physician's prescription and/or referral for appropriate care. It also suggests that the problem may go beyond that of physicians to include other healthcare practitioners.

Provider Cultural Competency and Healthcare Disparities

Cultural competence has been defined as a set of behaviors, attitudes, and policies that enable effective work in cross-cultural situations (Anderson, Scrimshaw, Fullilove, Fielding, & Normand, 2003). Culture refers to integrated patterns of behavior including language, thoughts, customs, and beliefs of religious, ethnic, or social groups (Anderson et al.). Competency refers to the capacity to function effectively as an individual within the context of cultural beliefs, beliefs and needs of consumers, and their communities (Anderson et al.). Interest in the role of cultural competency continues to grow as does the realization of the increasing diversity of the US populace. While the need for cultural competency is most often discussed as a need of providers, health care and medical practice are being provided increasingly by a team or mix of individuals. Because minorities are significantly underrepresented in the healthcare workforce, the need for cultural competency is heightened, but will only occur with the support, and in the context, of the broader healthcare system (Brach & Fraser, 2000). In addition, if long-term institutionalization is to occur, cultural competency will need to be addressed at the institutional level. As such, this section will briefly outline the issue of cultural competency only as it relates to providers. The concept will be more broadly developed in the chapter on healthcare systems.

Much of the cultural competency literature is focused on cultural awareness, knowledge attitudes, and skills of providers. Indeed, the potential need for this focus is suggested by studies that document significant proportions of minorities reporting that they believe they would have received better care if they had been seen by a doctor of a different race or ethnicity (Collins et al., 2002). As many as 16% of African-Americans and 18% of Hispanics indicate that they had been treated with disrespect during a healthcare visit. The reasons for these beliefs were often attributed to communications-related factors such as being spoken to rudely, talked down to, or otherwise ignored (Collins et al.). Asian-Americans are least likely to feel that their doctors understand their beliefs and values and they are the most likely group to report that their doctors looked down on them (Collins et al.). Interestingly though, one-third of all adults report using complementary or alternative therapies and remedies within the past 2 years, with the highest rates being reported among White adults (Collins et al.). On the other hand, African-Americans, Hispanics, and Asians who use alternative remedies are less likely to tell their doctors about it than White patients (Collins et al.). Finally, in a recent classic study by Lillie-Blanton et al., a representative sample of US citizens were asked to indicate their thoughts regarding whether the average African-American receives lower quality care, about the same quality care, or higher quality care as the average White person? The results indicated that while a majority of White Americans (68%) believed that African-Americans receive the same or higher quality care than most Whites, most African-Americans (64%) believed that they receive lower quality care than most Whites (Lillie-Blanton, Brodie, Rowland, Altman, & McIntosh, 2000).

Summary

From the discussion above it can be seen that culture and ethnicity often create unique patterns of beliefs, behaviors, and perceptions regarding health, illness, providers, patients, and the provision of care. These patterns influence the provider's ability or likelihood in recognizing certain patient symptoms. They also influence what patients choose to tell providers about their health. These factors impact provider interpretations of symptoms and patient adherence to therapy (Anderson et al., 2003). The evidence also suggests that racial and ethnic minority patients do not receive the appropriate and recommended care as clinically similar White patients for those services that require provider referral. As such, the evidence suggests that several factors related specifically to providers likely contribute to differential outcomes and the persistence of healthcare disparities.

References

Anderson, L., Scrimshaw, S., Fullilove, M., Fielding, J., & Normand, J. (2003). Culturally competent healthcare systems: A systematic review. *American Journal of Preventive Medicine, 24*, 68–79.

Bernabei, R., Gambassi, G., Lapane, K., Landi, F., Gatsonis, C., Dunlop, R., et al. (1998). Management of pain in elderly patients with cancer. SAGE Study Group. Systematic assessment of geriatric drug use via epidemiology. *JAMA: The Journal of the American Medical Association, 279*, 1877–1882.

Brach, C., & Fraser, I. (2000). Can cultural competency reduce racila and ethnic disparities? A review and conceptual model. *Medical Care Research and Review, 57*, 181–217.

Brennan, T. A., Hebert, L. E., Laird, N. M., Lawthers, A., Thorpe, K. E., Leape, L. L., et al. (1991). Hospital characteristics associated with adverse events and substandard care. *JAMA: The Journal of the American Medical Association, 265*, 3265–3269.

Brennan, T. A., Leape, L. L., Laird, N. M., Hebert, L., Localio, A. R., Lawthers, A. G., et al. (1991). Incidence of adverse events and negligence in hospitalized patients. Results of the Harvard Medical Practice Study I. *The New England Journal of Medicine, 324*, 370–376.

Brennan, T. A., Leape, L. L., Laird, N. M., Localio, A. R., & Hiatt, H. H. (1990). Incidence of adverse events and negligent care in hospitalized patients. *Transactions of the Association of American Physicians, 103*, 137–144.

Charles, H., Good, C., Hanusa, B., Chang, C., & Whittle, J. (2003). Racial Differences in adherence to cardiac medications. *Journal of the National Medical Association, 95*, 22.

Cleeland, C. S., Gonin, R., Baez, L., Loehrer, P., & Pandya, K. J. (1997). Pain and treatment of pain in minority patients with cancer. The Eastern Cooperative Oncology Group Minority Outpatient Pain Study. *Annals of Internal Medicine, 127*, 813–816.

Collins, K. S., Hughes, D. L., Doty, M. M., Ives, B. L., Edwards, J. N., & Tenney, K. (2002). *Diverse communities, common concerns: Assessing health care quality for minority Americans* (Rep. No. 523). The Commonwealth Fund.

Gregory, P. C., LaVeist, T. A., & Simpson, C. (2006). Racial disparities in access to cardiac rehabilitation. *American Journal of Physical Medicine and Rehabilitation, 85*, 705–710.

Hill, M., Bone, L., Kim, M., Miller, D., Dennison, C., & Levine, D. (1999). Barriers to hypertension care and control in young urban black men. *American Journal of Hypertension, 12*, 951–958.

Kaplan, S. H., Greenfield, S., & Ware, J. E., Jr. (1989). Assessing the effects of physician–patient interactions on the outcomes of chronic disease. *Medical Care, 27*, S110–S127.

LaVeist, T. A. (2002). *Race, Ethnicity and Health.* San Francisco: Jose-Bass.

LaVeist, T. A., Arthur, M., Morgan, A., Plantholt, S., & Rubinstein, M. (2003). Explaining racial differences in receipt of coronary angiography: The role of physician referral and physician specialty. *Medical Care Research and Review, 60*, 453–467.

Leape, L. L., Brennan, T. A., Laird, N., Lawthers, A. G., Localio, A. R., Barnes, B. A., et al. (1991). The nature of adverse events in hospitalized patients. Results of the Harvard Medical Practice Study II. *The New England Journal of Medicine, 324*, 377–384.

Lillie-Blanton, M., Brodie, M., Rowland, D., Altman, D., & McIntosh, M. (2000). Race, ethnicity, and the health care system: Public perceptions and experiences. *Medical Care Research and Review, 57*(Suppl. 1), 218–235.

Morrison, R. S., Wallenstein, S., Natale, D. K., Senzel, R. S., & Huang, L. L. (2000). "We don't carry that" – Failure of pharmacies in predominantly nonwhite neighborhoods to stock opioid analgesics. *The New England Journal of Medicine, 342*, 1023–1026.

Mumford, E., Schlesinger, H. J., & Glass, G. V. (1982). The effect of psychological intervention on recovery from surgery and heart attacks: An analysis of the literature. *American Journal of Public Health, 72*, 141–151.

Ong, L. M., de Haes, J. C., Hoos, A. M., & Lammes, F. B. (1995). Doctor–patient communication: A review of the literature. *Social Science & Medicine, 40*, 903–918.

Orth, J. E., Stiles, W. B., Scherwitz, L., Hennrikus, D., & Vallbona, C. (1987). Patient exposition and provider explanation in routine interviews and hypertensive patients' blood pressure control. *Health Psychology: Official journal of the Division of Health Psychology, American Psychological Association, 6*, 29–42.

Rose, L., Kim, M., Dennison, C., & Hill, M. (2000). The context of adherence for African-Americans with high blood pressure. *Journal of Advanced Nursing, 32*, 587–594.

Roter, D. L. (1989). Which facets of communication have strong effects on outcomes – A metanalysis. In M. Stewart, & D. L. Roter (Eds.), *Communicating with medical patients.* Newbury Park, CA: Sage Publications.

Roter, D., & Hall, J. (1993). *Doctors talking with patients, patients talking with doctors.* London: Auburn House.

Roter, D. L., Hall, J. A., & Katz, N. R. (1987). Relations between physicians' behaviors and analogue patients' satisfaction, recall, and impressions. *Medical Care, 25*, 437–451.

Sarver, J., & Baker, D. W. (2000). Effect of language barriers on follow-up appointments after an emergency department visit. *Journal of General Internal Medicine, 15*, 256–264.

Schulman, K. A., Berlin, J. A., Harless, W., Kerner, J. F., Sistrunk, S., Gersh, B. J., et al. (1999). The effect of race and sex on physicians' recommendations for cardiac catheterization. *The New England Journal of Medicine, 340*, 618–626.

Smedley, B. D., Stith, A. Y., & Nelson, A. R. (2003). *Unequal treatment: Confronting racial and ethnic disparities in healthcare.* Washington, DC: National Academy Press.

Williams, S., Weinman, J., & Dale, J. (1998). Doctor–patient communication and patient satisfaction: A review. *Family Practice, 15*, 480–492.

3
Patient Factors in Healthcare Disparities

Michael Christopher Gibbons

Access to Care/Insurance Status

A significant literature exists regarding the role of patient factors in the causation of racial and ethnic healthcare disparities. Major determinants include healthcare access/insurance status, language dominance, patient health literacy, mistrust of providers, patient preferences and refusal of treatment, and race-based biophysiologic difference. Racial and ethnic disparities in access to medical care are well known among health service researchers (Andrulis, 1998). Previous research has shown consistently that people without health insurance are less likely to receive health care in a timely manner and have lower levels of health services utilization (Andrulis; Bradbury, Golec, & Steen, 2001). In addition, most studies conclude that members of minority ethnic groups are less likely to have insurance and more likely to have insurance related healthcare access problems than Whites (Bradbury et al.; Fiscella, Franks, Doescher, & Saver, 2002; Gaskin & Hoffman, 2000; Hogue, Hargraves, & Collins, 2000; Mayberry, Mili, & Ofili, 2000; Monheit & Vistnes, 2000; Waidmann & Rajan, 2000; Weinick, Jacobs, Stone, Ortega, & Burstin, 2004; Weinick & Krauss, 2000; Weinick, Zuvekas, & Cohen, 2000).

Perhaps the most well studied is the relationship of insurance status and medical care for heart disease. Publicly insured individuals are less likely than privately insured persons to receive cardiovascular procedures (Carlisle, Leake, & Shapiro, 1995, 1997a, 1997b; Wenneker, Weissman, & Epstein, 1990). Racial differences in use of cardiovascular procedures have been reported among publicly insured persons, but not among those with private insurance (Carlisle et al., 1997b). Finally, differences between ethnic groups in terms of care for cardiac disease narrow when persons obtain adequate insurance coverage, such as eligibility for Medicare (Hargraves & Hadley, 2003).

Racial and ethnic disparities in access to care, however, are not fully explained by differences in sociodemographics or health status (Weinick & Krauss, 2000; Zuvekas & Taliaferro, 2003). In fact, these problems persist even among those covered by insurance, although they are more pronounced among persons who lack insurance or live in areas with high levels of poverty (Andrulis, 1997, 1998; Fiscella et al., 2002).

Language Dominance

Racial and ethnic disparities in health care have been documented among individuals who do not speak English as their primary language. Much of the work in this area has evaluated potential effects within the Hispanic community. Hispanics, like African-Americans and other minority groups are at increased risk of poor health status, a higher incidence of diabetes, HIV, and cervical cancer (Berkman & Gurland, 1998; Black, Ray, & Markides, 1999; Burke et al., 1999; Gilliland, Hunt, & Key, 1998; Obiri, Fordyce, Singh, & Forlenza, 1998; Parker, Davis, Wingo, Ries, & Heath, 1998). In addition individuals who do not speak English are less likely to have a regular healthcare provider (Kirkman-Liff & Mondragon, 1991) and they have lower rates of utilization of preventive services (Woloshin, Bickell, Schwartz, Gany, & Welch, 1995; Woloshin, Schwartz, Katz, & Welch, 1997) and are at higher risk for drug complications (Ghandi, 2000). The data are conflicting in terms of healthcare utilization with some studies indicating higher utilization (Hampers, Cha, Gutglass, Binns, & Krug, 1999) while others indicate lower utilization rates among non-English speakers (Guendelman & Wagner, 2000; Weinick et al., 2004).

In general, Hispanics, like African-Americans are less likely to be insured and as such may have more limited access to healthcare providers and services (Monheit & Vistnes, 2000; Weinick et al., 2000, 2004). Language concordance refers to the notion of doctors and patients who speak the same language and is essential for obtaining an accurate medical history, assessing patient beliefs, and for establishing an empathetic doctor–patient relationship (Smedley, Stith, & Nelson, 2003). Communication failures can lead to providers misunderstanding their patients' concerns, misdiagnosing their patients' problems, and thereby lead to unnecessary testing (Smedley et al.) or failure to obtain needed testing. On the other hand, poor communication can lead to patients' misunderstanding the actions or motives of their doctors, lead to nonadherance and contribute to patient lack of desire or unwillingness to return for appropriate follow-up visits with their providers (Smedley et al.).

It is important to note that communication problems are not limited to patients and doctors who speak different languages. Significant communication barriers may exist in so-called language concordant physician–patient encounters where the doctor and the patients both speak English. In the US, approximately 14 million people have Limited English Proficiency (LEP). LEP problems can be related to patient literacy levels (discussed below). Certain ethnic or cultural factors including linguistic accents or the use of idioms or the use of regional vernacular, may at times pose communication challenges that manifest within the context of the clinical encounter. For example a young African-American physician from New York City may at times experience difficulty in understanding and communicating with an elderly white patient from the bayous of Mississippi.

Several researchers have evaluated the efficacy of professional vs. untrained interpreters, patient interpreter preferences, patient satisfaction, and the ethical implications of various types of language interpreters (Elderkin-Thompson, Silver,

& Waitzkin, 2001; Flores, 2005; Flores, Laws, et al., 2003; Flores, Rabke-Verani, Pine, & Sabharwal, 2002; Jacobs et al., 2001; Phelan & Parkman, 1995). Generally these studies recommend using professional interpreters to improve the quality of health care delivered to both limited English proficient individuals and alternate language dominate individuals. Using trained indigenous workers as interpreters is preferable to family members or other untrained individuals due to significant ethical problems and increased risk of interpretational errors with nonprofessional interpreters (Elderkin-Thompson et al.; Flores; Flores, Laws, et al.; Jacobs et al.; Phelan & Parkman).

Health Literacy

Health literacy is defined as the ability to read and comprehend health-related materials (Baker, 1999). The results of the National Adult Literacy Survey reveal that approximately 40 million Americans, fully 25% of the US population, suffer from inadequate literacy (Weiss & Coyne, 1997). To complicate matters further, 80% of English- and Spanish-speaking patients over the age of 60 were low literate (Gazmararian et al., 1999), while still other studies document a disproportionate prevalence of low literacy among low-income, urban populations (Williams et al., 1995).

Low-literate patients are less likely to understand hospital discharge instructions or know essential information about diseases including hypertension, diabetes, and asthma (Baker, 1999). For example, low-literate asthmatic patients are less likely to know how to use their metered dose inhalers to control or prevent an asthma attack (Baker).

Many health literacy studies rely on the number of school years completed as the sole measure of literacy (Baker, 1999). However, other factors including English language proficiency and age influence health literacy. Measuring the number of years of school, measures education completed. Health literacy on the other hand reflects what was learned during those years and an individual's ability to comprehend new material (Baker).

More than 200 papers have been published since the early 1990s on the topic of health literacy. Most, however, focused on the gap between patient literacy levels and the required literacy levels needed to read most health materials (Roter, Rudd, & Comings, 1998). As a consequence, most interventions developed employ the utilization of simplified health materials and visual aids or other provider strategies to improve patient recall and understanding (Roter et al.).

In terms of physiologic outcomes related to literacy barriers, among HIV patients, patients who report nonadherance to HAART and have lower health literacy rates also are more likely to have significantly lower CD4 cell counts and significantly less likely to have an undetectable viral load when compared with higher literate and adherent patients (Ong, de Haes, Hoos, & Lammes, 1995). Higher hospitalization rates have also been linked to low patient literacy (Baker,

1999). The biologic mechanisms responsible for these observations have not been definitively characterized, although psychoneuroimmunological mechanisms and pathways generally described by social network theory have been hypothesized (Kaplan, Greenfield, & Ware, 1989; Roter & Hall, 1993).

In a study specifically designed to examine the effect of English fluency on health services utilization, Fiscella reported that healthcare utilization patterns for English-speaking Hispanic patients did not differ from patterns of non-Hispanic Whites. However, Spanish-speaking Hispanics were significantly less likely than English-speaking Hispanics to have had a physician visit, mental health visit, or influenza vaccination. African-American patients also exhibited significantly lower rates of influenza vaccination and a mental health visit after adjustment for predisposing, enabling, and need factors (Fiscella et al., 2002).

Few studies of language barriers evaluate financial data or cost implications. One available study was conducted in a large urban Hispanic population with available interpreters. Language barriers were defined as a family English language proficiency level that posed a barrier to the treating physician. This study revealed that when doctor–family language barriers exist, patients experience higher charges ($38 per patient) due to more diagnostic testing and approximately 20 min longer ER stays compared to similarly acute patients without family–doctor language barriers (Roter et al., 1998).

Mistrust of Medical Providers or the Healthcare System

Some minorities express higher levels of mistrust of providers and the healthcare system than Whites. It has been suggested that this mistrust stems in part from historic breeches of trust that have occurred within the medical system. Most notably the Public Health Services study of Syphillis among African-Americans which was conducted from 1932 to 1972 in Tuskegee, Alabama is most often cited (Freimuth et al., 2001; Gamble, 1997; Shavers, Lynch, & Burmeister, 2000; Smedley et al., 2003; Thomas & Curran, 1999; Thomas & Quinn, 1991). In this study of the natural history of Syphillis, 399 African-American men with latent syphillis were followed, but not treated for their disease. Individuals enrolled in the study did not give informed consent and were not informed of their diagnosis (Gamble). Many African-Americans, however, believe that the mistrust predated public revelations about the Tuskegee study. Rather they contend that the historic mistrust of the medical community among African-Americans should be seen in a broader historical and social context, where several factors have and continue to influence African-Americans' attitudes toward the healthcare system (Gamble).

Breeches of trust are not limited, however, to African-Americans. In 1955 military medical researchers attempted to study the role of the thyroid gland in acclimatization of humans to cold weather. In this study, radioactive iodine was given to 102 American-Indians and 19 military personnel. Forty years later, questions were raised regarding the selection process, their understanding of the research, and the risks involved. A recent comprehensive study of the event by the Institute of Medicine concluded that information on the nature of the radioactive tracer used in the study was not fully disclosed to all participants, and they were not completely informed about the nature and risks of the experiments. In addition minor children were used without adequate parental consent. Perhaps most troubling is the fact that few of the Alaska Natives understood that they were participating in research; instead, most thought they were receiving needed medical treatment (Institute of Medicine, 1996).

This legacy of mistrust among racial and ethic minorities may discourage some minorities from seeking care appropriately, or from consenting to certain therapies (Smedley et al., 2003). It has led to the belief among many minorities that they are treated differently in the healthcare system solely because of their race and that this difference in treatment is a reflection of a broader devaluation of the lives of minority Americans by society (Gamble, 1997). Among undocumented Hispanics and immigrants this mistrust may stem from fear of deportation (Canlas, 1999). The undocumented often harbor the constant fear of being investigated by authorities. Healthcare workers may be viewed as extensions of government agencies. As a result the fear of deportation and perceived threats to personal security and well-being are very real. There is often a great reluctance on the part of undocumented persons especially within the Latino community to seek health care because they fear investigation and exposure of their illegal status (Canlas).

Patient experiences of real or perceived bias or discrimination may inhibit minority patients' motivation to participate actively and fully in the healthcare encounter (Smedley et al., 2003). Indeed, it has been shown that African-American patients are more likely than Whites to report having experienced discrimination during a healthcare visit (Smedley et al.). They are also less likely than White patients to believe that doctors treat African-Americans the same as White patients. These findings corroborate the fact that African-Americans are more likely to believe that racial discrimination in the doctor's office is a commonplace event (LaVeist, Nickerson, & Bowie, 2000) and are significantly more likely than Whites to mistrust the healthcare system (LaVeist et al.).

Patient Preferences and Refusal of Treatment

It has been suggested that patient refusal of physician recommendations may contribute to racial and ethnic disparities in health care. There is a paucity of experimental data evaluating this premise in the scientific literature. Among the few studies that do exist, the evidence is somewhat mixed. A few studies do suggest that African-American patients may be more likely than White patients to refuse invasive procedures like surgery or coronary bypass procedures, however, some of these same studies show that physicians recommend these treatments more often to their White patients in comparison to their Black patients. As such, physician bias is contributing to observed variations even before patients have the opportunity to make a choice (Smedley et al., 2003). In contrast, several studies find no difference in refusal rates between Whites and minorities or if refusal rates do differ, the magnitude of the observed differences cannot fully explain the documented disparities (Smedley et al.). Unfortunately the causes of these increase refusal rates have not been well studied or characterized. Given the findings of higher levels of mistrust, lower satisfaction with care, and greater likelihood of experiencing discrimination in the healthcare setting by African-Americans and other racial minorities, the higher refusal rate may be related to these broader perceptions of the healthcare system (Smedley et al.).

Biologic Differences

Although the subject of significant debate, biologic factors may contribute to the occurrence of racial and ethnic disparities in health care. In respect to the cardio-vascular diseases for example, recognized clinical differences in response to pharmacotherapy occur within many homogenous and nonhomogenous populations (Sowers, Ferdinand, Bakris, & Douglas, 2002). Scientific data suggest that response variability to hypertensive medications occur in both African-American and White populations (Exner, Dries, Domanski, & Cohn, 2001; Sareli et al., 2001; Weir, Gray, Paster, & Saunders, 1995; Yancy et al., 2001). In addition among some minority populations, especially African-Americans, there appears to exist an enhanced sensitivity to dietary sodium intake. Thus at a given level of dietary sodium, African-American patients may be at higher risk of developing hypertension than Whites. In addition, other factors including cardiovascular reactivity, vascular resistance, prevalence of left ventricular hypertrophy (LVH), insulin resistance, and hyperinsulinemia may differ among African-Americans and thus, may also impact the development of disparities in hypertension and cardiovascular disease (Chapman et al., 1999; McFarlane, Banerji, & Sowers, 2001; Sowers, 1998; Sowers, Epstein, & Frohlich, 2001; Sowers, Ferdinand, et al.). These complex biologic factors and social realities are interrelated and difficult to separate. In the future, studies that attempt to elucidate the biologic mechanisms underlying the socially oriented determinants of hypertension and CVD will be needed.

Sociocultural and Behavioral Factors

Increasingly various sociocultural factors have been suggested as possible contributors to racial and ethnic disparities in health care. For example culturally oriented diets and body appearance norms are being recognized as contributors to the problems of observed racial and ethnic disparities in obesity, hypertension, and diabetes rates (Watkins, 2004). African-American perceptions of "desirable" weight appear to be higher than that of White women. This belief may be an important factor in the finding that African-American women have the highest levels of obesity in the US. This in turn may contribute to higher levels of hypertension and diabetes seen among this group (Watkins).

The belief that health outcomes are ordained of God and therefore cannot be changed, also referred to as fatalism, has been documented as a cultural factor among African-Americans (Kressin & Petersen, 2001). It has been suggested that this belief may impact decision making among African-American patients and contribute to hypertensive disparities (Ferguson et al., 1998).

Culturally determined myths may be important in the genesis of hypertension disparities. Hill reported that AA men incorrectly described being healthy as being symptom free and as a result, self-adjusted their medication usage depending on the existence of "symptoms." In addition these men considered buying antihypertensive medications a luxury, because of their high cost. They also thought that seeking help for hypertension was a sign of weakness or laziness (Rose, Kim, Dennison, & Hill, 2000). These attitudes and beliefs may in part also be responsible for the finding of suboptimal medication adherence and inadequate self-monitoring of blood pressure among African-Americans (Chobanian et al., 2003). Unfortunately the scientific evidence indicates as many as 50% of newly diagnoses hypertensive discontinue use of prescribed meds within 1 year of diagnosis and up to 50% of the remaining patients do not take their medications as prescribed (Friday, 1999). As such, issues of poor medication adherence and inadequate self-monitoring are problems in the entire population but are especially problematic among African-American patients (Artinian, Washington, & Templin, 2001; Friday; Hill et al., 1999; Rose et al.).

Summary

In summary, several patient-related factors may contribute to the development of healthcare disparities. Access to care and insurance status are often considered together and so related to each other, that the effects of each are hard to separate. Both, whether alone or together have been shown to be less likely among racial and ethnic minorities. Not having health insurance or having inadequate access to care has been consistently been found to be associated with inappropriate healthcare utilization, underutilization, longer lengths of stay as well as poorer health outcomes among racial and ethnic minorities. While poor access to care and lack of health insurance are problems most likely to be found among the poor, access-related healthcare disparities persist even among racial and ethnic minorities who are insured, well educated, and employed.

Several languages related factors are also important. The most obvious of these is the inability to speak English. Non-English speakers who typically are Hispanics and other immigrants have poorer access to care and are at increased risk for poor health outcomes than Whites. The use of medical interpreters is one possible way to help address this issue although providers and healthcare systems often use less appropriate family members and friends due to the limited availability of these professions within the healthcare system. Health literacy is a related language problem that affects an estimated 25% of the US population. The poor, racial, and ethnic minorities, and those living in the urban inner city are at highest risk for being poorly health literate. Poor health literacy is thought to influence a patient's ability to understand his or her medical condition and or comply with the provider's instructions and recommendations. Mistrust of the healthcare system is another factor among many racial and ethnic minorities that may influence the development of healthcare disparities. This mistrust is rooted in historic and contemporary breeches of trust that have led many minorities to believe that their lives are relatively devalued within the broader society. Mistrust is also a significant factor among undocumented immigrants. Because of fears of deportation and the perception that healthcare providers may work as an arm of the immigration service many undocumented immigrants may be unwilling to seek care appropriately. While there is some evidence to suggest that patient preferences among racial and ethnic minority patients may disagree with the recommendations of their providers, this difference is generally not sufficient to explain the level of disparities that have been documented. Finally, although it is still the subject of significant debate, it is possible that certain biologic factors may contribute to the development of healthcare disparities. Much more work needs to be done to elucidate the existence of these biological differences and the relationship of any identified differences to the genesis of healthcare disparities.

References

Andrulis, D. P. (1997). The urban health penalty: New dimensions and directions in inner city health care. In *Inner city health care*. Philadelphia: American College of Physicians.

Andrulis, D. P. (1998). Access to care is the centerpiece in the elimination of socioeconomic disparities in health. *Annals of Internal Medicine, 129*, 412–416.

Artinian, N. T., Washington, O. G., & Templin, T. N. (2001). Effects of home telemonitoring and community-based monitoring on blood pressure control in urban African Americans: A pilot study. *Heart Lung, 30*, 191–199.

Baker, D. W. (1999). Reading between the lines: Deciphering the connections between literacy and health. *Journal of General Internal Medicine, 14*, 315–317.

Berkman, C. S., & Gurland, B. J. (1998). The relationship between ethnoracial group and functional level in older persons. *Ethnicity & Health, 3*, 175–188.

Black, S. A., Ray, L. A., & Markides, K. S. (1999). The prevalence and health burden of self-reported diabetes in older Mexican Americans: Findings from the Hispanic established populations for epidemiologic studies of the elderly. *American Journal of Public Health, 89*, 546–552.

Bradbury, R. C., Golec, J. H., & Steen, P. M. (2001). Comparing uninsured and privately insured hospital patients: Admission severity, health outcomes and resource use. *Health Services Management Research, 14*, 203–210.

Burke, J. P., Williams, K., Gaskill, S. P., Hazuda, H. P., Haffner, S. M., & Stern, M. P. (1999). Rapid rise in the incidence of type 2 diabetes from 1987 to 1996: Results from the San Antonio Heart Study. *Archives of Internal Medicine, 159*, 1450–1456.

Canlas, L. G. (1999). Issues of health care mistrust in East Harlem. *Mount Sinai Journal of Medicine, 66*, 257–258.

Carlisle, D. M., Leake, B. D., & Shapiro, M. F. (1995). Racial and ethnic differences in the use of invasive cardiac procedures among cardiac patients in Los Angeles County, 1986 through 1988. *American Journal of Public Health, 85*, 352–356.

Carlisle, D. M., Leake, B. D., & Shapiro, M. F. (1997a). African Americans and Latinos are least likely to receive high-tech heart treatments. *Policy Brief (UCLA Center for Health Policy Research)*, 1–4.

Carlisle, D. M., Leake, B. D., & Shapiro, M. F. (1997b). Racial and ethnic disparities in the use of cardiovascular procedures: Associations with type of health insurance. *American Journal of Public Health, 87*, 263–267.

Chapman, J. N., Mayet, J., Chang, C. L., Foale, R. A., Thom, S. A., & Poulter, N. R. (1999). Ethnic differences in the identification of left ventricular hypertrophy in the hypertensive patient. *American Journal of Hypertension, 12*, 437–442.

Chobanian, A. V., Bakris, G. L., Black, H. R., Cushman, W. C., Green, L. A., Izzo, J. L., Jr., et al. (2003). The seventh report of the joint national committee on prevention, detection, evaluation, and treatment of high blood pressure: The JNC 7 report. *JAMA: The Journal of the American Medical Association, 289*, 2560–2572.

Elderkin-Thompson, V., Silver, R. C., & Waitzkin, H. (2001). When nurses double as interpreters: A study of Spanish-speaking patients in a US primary care setting. *Social Science & Medicine, 52*, 1343–1358.

Exner, D. V., Dries, D. L., Domanski, M. J., & Cohn, J. N. (2001). Lesser response to angiotensin-converting-enzyme inhibitor therapy in black as compared with white patients with left ventricular dysfunction. *The New England Journal of Medicine, 344*, 1351–1357.

Ferguson, J. A., Weinberger, M., Westmoreland, G. R., Mamlin, L. A., Segar, D. S., Greene, J. Y., et al. (1998). Racial disparity in cardiac decision making: Results from patient focus groups. *Archives of Internal Medicine, 158*, 1450–1453.

Fiscella, K., Franks, P., Doescher, M. P., & Saver, B. G. (2002). Disparities in health care by race, ethnicity, and language among the insured: Findings from a national sample. *Medical Care, 40*, 52–59.

Flores, G. (2005). The impact of medical interpreter services on the quality of health care: A systematic review. *Medical Care Research and Review, 62*, 255–299.

Flores, G., Laws, M. B., Mayo, S. J., Zuckerman, B., Abreu, M., Medina, L., et al. (2003). Errors in medical interpretation and their potential clinical consequences in pediatric encounters. *Pediatrics, 111*, 6–14.

Flores, G., Rabke-Verani, J., Pine, W., & Sabharwal, A. (2002). The importance of cultural and linguistic issues in the emergency care of children. *Pediatric Emergency Care, 18*, 271–284.

Freimuth, V. S., Quinn, S. C., Thomas, S. B., Cole, G., Zook, E., & Duncan, T. (2001). African Americans' views on research and the Tuskegee Syphilis study. *Social Science & Medicine, 52*, 797–808.

Friday, G. H. (1999). Antihypertensive medication compliance in African-American stroke patients: Behavioral epidemiology and interventions. *Neuroepidemiology, 18*, 223–230.

Gamble, V. N. (1997). Under the shadow of Tuskegee: African Americans and health care. *American Journal of Public Health, 87*, 1773–1778.

Gaskin, D. J., & Hoffman, C. (2000). Racial and ethnic differences in preventable hospitalizations across 10 states. *Medical Care Research and Review, 57*(Suppl. 1), 85–107.

Gazmararian, J. A., Baker, D. W., Williams, M. V., Parker, R. M., Scott, T. L., Green, D. C., et al. (1999). Health literacy among medicare enrollees in a managed care organization. *JAMA: The Journal of the American Medical Association, 281*, 545–551.

Ghandi, R. (2000). IDSA update from the city of brotherly love. The *Hopkins HIV Report, 12*, 1, 4, 11.

Gilliland, F. D., Hunt, W. C., & Key, C. R. (1998). Trends in the survival of American Indian, Hispanic, and Non-Hispanic white cancer patients in New Mexico and Arizona, 1969–1994. *Cancer, 82*, 1769–1783.

Guendelman, S., & Wagner, T. H. (2000). Health services utilization among Latinos and white non-Latinos: Results from a national survey. *Journal of Health Care for the Poor and Underserved, 11*, 179–194.

Hampers, L. C., Cha, S., Gutglass, D. J., Binns, H. J., & Krug, S. E. (1999). Language barriers and resource utilization in a pediatric emergency department. *Pediatrics, 103*, 1253–1256.

Hargraves, J. L., & Hadley, J. (2003). The contribution of insurance coverage and community resources to reducing racial/ethnic disparities in access to care. *Health Service Research, 38*, 809–829.

Hill, M., Bone, L., Kim, M., Miller, D., Dennison, C., & Levine, D. (1999). Barriers to hypertension care and control in young urban black men. *American Journal of Hypertension, 12*, 951–958.

Hogue, C., Hargraves, M., & Collins, K. (2000). *Minority health in America: Findings and policy implications from the commonwealth fund minority health survey*. Baltimore: Johns Hopkins University Press.

Institute of Medicine. (1996). *The Arctic aeromedical laboratory's thyroid function study: A radiological risk and ethical analysis*. Washington, DC: National Academy Press.

Jacobs, E. A., Lauderdale, D. S., Meltzer, D., Shorey, J. M., Levinson, W., & Thisted, R. A. (2001). Impact of interpreter services on delivery of health care to limited-English-proficient patients. *Journal of General Internal Medicine, 16*, 468–474.

Kaplan, S. H., Greenfield, S., & Ware, J. E., Jr. (1989). Assessing the effects of physician–patient interactions on the outcomes of chronic disease. *Medical Care, 27*, S110–S127.

Kirkman-Liff, B., & Mondragon, D. (1991). Language of interview: Relevance for research of southwest Hispanics. *American Journal of Public Health, 81*, 1399–1404.

Kressin, N. R., & Petersen, L. A. (2001). Racial differences in the use of invasive cardiovascular procedures: Review of the literature and prescription for future research. *Annals of Internal Medicine, 135*, 352–366.

LaVeist, T. A., Nickerson, K. J., & Bowie, J. V. (2000). Attitudes about racism, medical mistrust, and satisfaction with care among African American and white cardiac patients. *Medical Care Research and Review, 57*(Suppl. 1), 146–161.

Mayberry, R. M., Mili, F., & Ofili, E. (2000). Racial and ethnic differences in access to medical care. *Medical Care Research and Review, 57*(Suppl. 1), 108–145.

McFarlane, S. I., Banerji, M., & Sowers, J. R. (2001). Insulin resistance and cardiovascular disease. *Journal of Clinical Endocrinology and Metabolism, 86*, 713–718.

Monheit, A. C., & Vistnes, J. P. (2000). Race/ethnicity and health insurance status: 1987 and 1996. *Medical Care Research and Review, 57*(Suppl. 1), 11–35.

Obiri, G. U., Fordyce, E. J., Singh, T. P., & Forlenza, S. (1998). Effect of HIV/AIDS versus other causes of death on premature mortality in New York City, 1983–1994. *American Journal of Epidemiology, 147*, 840–845.

Ong, L. M., de Haes, J. C., Hoos, A. M., & Lammes, F. B. (1995). Doctor–patient communication: A review of the literature. *Social Science & Medicine, 40*, 903–918.

Parker, S. L., Davis, K. J., Wingo, P. A., Ries, L. A., & Heath, C. W., Jr. (1998). Cancer statistics by race and ethnicity. *CA-A Cancer Journal for Clinicians, 48*, 31–48.

Phelan, M., & Parkman, S. (1995). How to work with an interpreter. *British Medical Journal, 311*, 555–557.

Rose, L., Kim, M., Dennison, C., & Hill, M. (2000). The context of adherance for African-Americans with high blood pressure. *Journal of Advanced Nursing, 32*, 587–594.

Roter, D., & Hall, J. (1993). *Doctors talking with patients, patients talking with doctors*. London: Auburn House.

Roter, D. L., Rudd, R. E., & Comings, J. (1998). Patient literacy. A barrier to quality of care. *Journal of General Internal Medicine, 13*, 850–851.

Sareli, P., Radevski, I. V., Valtchanova, Z. P., Libhaber, E., Candy, G. P., Den Hond, E., et al. (2001). Efficacy of different drug classes used to initiate antihypertensive treatment in black subjects: Results of a randomized trial in Johannesburg, South Africa. *Archives of Internal Medicine, 161*, 965–971.

Shavers, V. L., Lynch, C. F., & Burmeister, L. F. (2000). Knowledge of the Tuskegee study and its impact on the willingness to participate in medical research studies. *Journal of the National Medical Association, 92,* 563–572.

Smedley, B. D., Stith, A. Y., & Nelson, A. R. (2003). *Unequal treatment: Confronting racial and ethnic disparities in healthcare.* Washington, DC: National Academy Press.

Sowers, J. R. (1998). Diabetes mellitus and cardiovascular disease in women. *Archives of Internal Medicine, 158,* 617–621.

Sowers, J. R., Epstein, M., & Frohlich, E. D. (2001). Diabetes, hypertension, and cardiovascular disease: An update. *Hypertension, 37,* 1053–1059.

Sowers, J. R., Ferdinand, K. C., Bakris, G. L., & Douglas, J. G. (2002). Hypertension-related disease in African Americans. Factors underlying disparities in illness and its outcome. *Postgraduate Medicine, 112,* 24–30, 33.

Thomas, S. B., & Curran, J. W. (1999). Tuskegee: From science to conspiracy to metaphor. *American Journal of the Medical Sciences, 317,* 1–4.

Thomas, S. B., & Quinn, S. C. (1991). The Tuskegee Syphilis Study, 1932 to 1972: Implications for HIV education and AIDS risk education programs in the black community. *American Journal of Public Health, 81,* 1498–1505.

Waidmann, T. A., & Rajan, S. (2000). Race and ethnic disparities in health care access and utilization: An examination of state variation. *Medical Care Research and Review, 57*(Suppl. 1), 55–84.

Watkins, L. O. (2004). Perspectives on coronary heart disease in African Americans. *Reviews in Cardiovascular Medicine, 5*(Suppl. 3), S3–S13.

Weinick, R. M., Jacobs, E. A., Stone, L. C., Ortega, A. N., & Burstin, H. (2004). Hispanic healthcare disparities: Challenging the myth of a monolithic Hispanic population. *Medical Care, 42,* 313–320.

Weinick, R. M., & Krauss, N. A. (2000). Racial/ethnic differences in children's access to care. *American Journal of Public Health, 90,* 1771–1774.

Weinick, R. M., Zuvekas, S. H., & Cohen, J. W. (2000). Racial and ethnic differences in access to and use of health care services, 1977 to 1996. *Medical Care Research and Review, 57*(Suppl. 1), 36–54.

Weir, M. R., Gray, J. M., Paster, R., & Saunders, E. (1995). Differing mechanisms of action of angiotensin-converting enzyme inhibition in black and white hypertensive patients. The Trandolapril Multicenter Study Group. *Hypertension, 26,* 124–130.

Weiss, B. D., & Coyne, C. (1997). Communicating with patients who cannot read. *The New England Journal of Medicine, 337,* 272–274.

Wenneker, M. B., Weissman, J. S., & Epstein, A. M. (1990). The association of payer with utilization of cardiac procedures in Massachusetts. *JAMA: The Journal of the American Medical Association, 264,* 1255–1260.

Williams, M. V., Parker, R. M., Baker, D. W., Parikh, N. S., Pitkin, K., Coates, W. C., et al. (1995). Inadequate functional health literacy among patients at two public hospitals. *JAMA: The Journal of the American Medical Association, 274,* 1677–1682.

Woloshin, S., Bickell, N. A., Schwartz, L. M., Gany, F., & Welch, H. G. (1995). Language barriers in medicine in the United States. *JAMA: The Journal of the American Medical Association, 273,* 724–728.

Woloshin, S., Schwartz, L. M., Katz, S. J., & Welch, H. G. (1997). Is language a barrier to the use of preventive services? *Journal of General Internal Medicine, 12,* 472–477.

Yancy, C. W., Fowler, M. B., Colucci, W. S., Gilbert, E. M., Bristow, M. R., Cohn, J. N., et al. (2001). Race and the response to adrenergic blockade with carvedilol in patients with chronic heart failure. *The New England Journal of Medicine, 344,* 1358–1365.

Zuvekas, S. H., & Taliaferro, G. S. (2003). Pathways to access: Health insurance, the health care delivery system, and racial/ethnic disparities, 1996–1999. *Health Affairs (Project Hope), 22,* 139–153.

4
Healthcare System Factors in Healthcare Disparities

Stephanie Chang and Michael Christopher Gibbons

Several aspects of the healthcare system have been postulated to impact patient care and outcomes, particularly among racial and ethnic minority groups (Smedley, Stith, & Nelson, 2003). These include, but are not limited to the organization, constitution and financing of the system as well as the ease of accessing services. Each of these factors will be discussed below.

Organization of Health Care

The fragmentary nature of the US healthcare system is in part responsible for a system ill-equipped to provide high quality care for every citizen. Recently investigators found that only 55% of participants in a large random sample of the US population received recommended health care. Similarly, the Institute of Medicine (IOM) found in its 1999 study of the healthcare system that 44,000–98,000 people die in US hospitals each year as a result of medical errors (Kohn, Corrigan, & Donaldson, 2000). In a March 2001 follow-up report, the Committee declared that the US healthcare system is plagued by serious quality problems resulting from an outmoded and inadequate delivery system, which is incapable of consistently providing high-quality care to its population (IOM Committee on Quality of Healthcare in America, 2001).

One factor that contributes to fragmentation and reduced quality relates to the multiple coverage options, offered by different health plans, which are accompanied by differing benefit packages. These packages often vary in terms of which providers a patient may choose. They also require patients to obtain varying amounts of preauthorization prior to obtaining care (Smedley et al., 2003). On an average, minority populations tend to have lower cost plans that restrict the use of healthcare services; Whites tend to have less restrictive plans (Smedley et al.). In part, this reality exists because among these plans, lower per capita budgets generally translate into fewer dollars to provide clinical services to patients (Smedley et al.).

Institutionally imposed physician financial and cost constraints may also foster disparate clinical practice patterns. This can be seen most graphically in the

Medicaid program where low reimbursement rates for doctors and hospitals are associated with the poor and many minorities being treated in "public" hospitals which maintain unique medical practice norms based on limited resources availability. In these facilities, hospital, human, diagnostic, and therapeutic resources tend to be lower and the care is more likely to be provided by students and physicians in specialty training (Smedley et al., 2003). Additionally Medicaid patients often have difficulty accessing private physicians and even being admitted to certain nonpublic hospitals where there often exist more highly trained providers and a greater availability of medical resources (Smedley et al.).

Finally, the US Department of Defense and the Veterans Affairs Systems maintain medical and healthcare systems which potentially offer more equitable care. The evidence, however, has been somewhat mixed. The Department of Defense system is specifically designed to offer universal access to all who qualify for services. Disparities in this system tend to be significantly attenuated or nonexistent (Smedley et al., 2003). The Veterans Administrations system, on the other hand, while comprehensive, is designed to significantly reduce financial barriers to care among military veterans. While the data is somewhat mixed, racial and ethnic disparities do seem to persist among veterans utilizing this system of care (Smedley et al.).

Access/Availability of Healthcare Providers and Technology

Recently, studies have emerged suggesting that where a person lives can itself have a significant impact on the level and quality of health care the patient receives (Baicker, Chandra, & Skinner, 2005; Baicker, Chandra, Skinner, & Wennberg, 2004; Fulcher & Kaukinen, 2004, 2005; Kaukinen & Fulcher, 2006; McPherson, Wennberg, Hovind, & Clifford, 1982; Susi & Mascarenhas, 2002; Vanasse et al., 2005). This is of importance because some minorities live in different areas than Whites' (Baicker et al., 2005). Several types of geography-related access barriers have been identified. Baicker, using Medicare claims data, found marked geographic differences in utilization of medical procedures between minorities and nonminorities. Some communities had very high levels of disparity while other communities had very low levels or no disparity at all (Baicker et al., 2005). This study also evaluated the distribution of providers and found that African-Americans tended to live in areas that have significantly higher levels of low quality providers (Baicker et al., 2005). In a related study, Baicker also found that a significant amount of geographic variability existed in relation to the availability of medical procedures. In other words, some regions had little or no racial disparities for a given procedure while other areas had significant amounts of variation for the same procedure (Baicker et al., 2004). As such, these authors concluded that geographic disparities in health care represented local phenomena more closely related to clinical or economic realities of the area rather than to race or ethnicity (Baicker et al., 2005).

In a large study of the quality of medical care provided in New York hospitals, Leape found disparities in patient iatrogenic injury resulting from substandard medical care (Brennan, Leape, et al., 1991; Brennan, Leape, Laird, Localio, & Hiatt, 1990; Leape et al., 1991). This was particularly evident in hospitals serving large proportions of minority patients (Brennan, Herbert, et al., 1991). However, when examining hospital quality and receipt of cardiac specialty procedures, disparities were found only among patients who came to the cardiac specialists via primary care physicians who worked at hospitals without cardiac specialty services. In other words, physicians working at hospitals without specialists tended not to refer patients to the hospitals with specialists. The underutilization of specialty services was particularly evident among uninsured patients (Leape, Hilborne, Bell, Kamberg, & Brook, 1999).

The utilization of cardiovascular medical devices such as the implantable cardioverter-defibrillator (ICD) and hospital-based procedures has increased markedly over the past 15 years (Schneider, Zaslavsky, & Epstein, 2002; Vining, Lurie, & Huang, 2003). There are indications, however, that these technologies are not used equally in different racial groups. Data suggest that the rate of ICD implantation among White patients consistently exceeds the rate among Blacks (Zipes et al., 2005). The root causes of these disparities may be related to geographic differences in the availability of medical technology. Black patients may be less likely to receive some medical technologies because they live in areas where the technologies are underutilized (Kurth et al., 2003) or not available (Baicker et al., 2004, 2005). Other data indicate that this discrepancy may be related to racial differences in travel patterns. For example, when the nearest hospitals did not include a high-technology hospital, Whites were more likely than Blacks to travel beyond those nearest hospitals to a high-technology hospital (Blustein & Weitzman, 1995). Similarly the actual difficulty a patient experiences in reaching a healthcare facility may impact the utilization of the facility. Low-income patients or those living in urban areas often commute via public transportation. For some this may be their only available form of transportation. Commuting via public or private transportation may significantly impact both the time involved and the ease of getting to a healthcare facility, regardless of the actual linear distance to a hospital. This in turn could contribute to differences in utilization patterns among certain groups of patients. Phibbs studied the correlation between linear straight line distance and travel time to a healthcare facility and found that while the correlation is often good, it may not hold, however, when studying specific hospitals, areas with very small numbers of hospitals, in urban environments characterized by high congestion, or when basing calculations on reliance on surface streets in areas with alternate public transportation resources (subways, commuter rail, taxi, shuttles) (Phibbs & Luft, 1995).

Finally, geographic disparities have also been found to contribute to lower rates of access to certain medicines and drugs. In a study evaluating the ease of filling prescriptions in New York city pharmacies, it was found that only 25% of pharmacies in predominately minority communities had sufficient supplies of certain pain medications. On the other hand, 72% of pharmacies in predominately

White communities carried adequate supplies of pain medicines (Morrison, Wallenstein, Natale, Senzel, & Huang, 2000).

Healthcare Workforce Diversity

Although the racial and ethnic diversity of the US continues to grow, the diversity of the health professions has remained essentially the same (Kennedy, 2005). African-Americans, Hispanics, and American-Indians currently account for approximately 6% of the nation's doctors and 7% of the nation's nurses and dentists despite comprising approximately one-third of the US population (Kennedy; Smedley et al., 2003). There is growing evidence that increasing diversity in the health professions has many benefits for the professionals themselves, their students, and their patients (Cone, Richardson, Todd, Betancourt, & Lowe, 2003).

Over the years, efforts to enhance the numbers of minority health professionals have been inhibited by a number of factors. Many minority students have poor early educational opportunities. Thus they are at a disadvantage when applying to health professional schools (Kennedy, 2005). In addition, these students are also more likely to face significant financial burdens that impact decisions regarding entry (Kennedy). Those minority students who do matriculate into professional school also face challenges with regard to academic appointments and promotions. Minority faculty comprises only 4.2% of faculty positions at US medical schools. Approximately 20% of these positions are located at three historically Black medical schools and three Puerto Rican medical schools (Betancourt & Maina, 2004). In addition, it has been shown that among medical school faculty White faculty are more likely to be promoted to senior academic rank than Asians, Hispanics, or African-Americans. This finding was not related to years of service nor other measures of academic productivity (Palepu et al., 1998). Rather it has been likened to the "glass ceiling" analogy that has been used to describe obstacles to female academic achievement (Cone et al., 2003). Minorities are also poorly represented in the medical specialties like cardiology, radiation oncology, and surgery (Cone et al.; Palepu et al.). This reality may also hold implications for referral practices among minority and disadvantaged patients.

In addition to physician workforce demographics, the need to enhance the diversity of the healthcare workforce is suggested by several other lines of evidence. Racial and ethnic minorities are four times more likely to receive care from non-White physicians than White physicians. Minority physicians on the other hand are much more likely to practice in minority or medically underserved communities (Cone et al., 2003; Smedley et al., 2003) and have greater percentages of minority and low-income patients who are covered by Medicaid (Gray & Stoddard, 1997; Keith, Bell, Swanson, & Williams, 1985; Komaromy et al., 1996; Lloyd, Johnson, & Mann, 1978).

It has been suggested that a more diverse healthcare workforce is one that is better equipped to train the next generation of providers who in fact will be caring for an increasingly diverse patient population (Smedley et al., 2003). Finally, increasing the diversity of the healthcare workforce may enhance doctor–patient communication and in turn enhance patient outcomes. Researchers have indeed shown that minority physicians are able to communicate more effectively with minority patients than do White physicians (Cooper-Patrick et al., 1999; Kaplan, Gandek, Greenfield, Rogers, & Ware, 1995). More effective communication will undoubtedly help strengthen patient and provider relationships. Evidence suggests that racially concordant patient–provider relationships (those in which the patient–provider shares a common racial or ethnic background) are associated with greater patient participation in the care process, higher patient satisfaction, and greater adherence to treatment (Cooper-Patrick et al.). Minority providers are generally more successful at recruiting minority patients into clinical trials. Enhancing the numbers of racial and ethnic minorities who participate in clinical research is critical to the healthcare system's ability to develop scientific advances and provide the highest quality medical services and products to every patient (Smedley et al.). Furthermore, racial and ethnic minority patients disproportionately receive their medical care in hospital emergency settings. Minority providers may be better able to tailor preventive health and primary care programs and services to meet the needs of minority patients and thereby enabling them to obtain more appropriate, less costly care in other clinical settings (Smedley et al.).

Healthcare Cultural Competency

Enhancing the cultural competence of the US healthcare system is increasingly advocated as one promising method to help address racial and ethnic healthcare disparities (Anderson, Scrimshaw, Fullilove, Fielding, & Normand, 2003; Betancourt, Green, & Carrillo, 2002; Betancourt & Maina, 2004; Brach & Fraser, 2000; Cone et al., 2003; Kennedy, 2005; Smedley et al., 2003). While cultural competence has been defined as a set of congruent attitudes, behaviors, and policies that come together in a system, agency, or among professionals that enables effective working in cross-cultural situations, the real idea behind cultural competency is that it is an explicit statement that a one-size-fits-all healthcare system cannot meet the needs of a diverse patient population (Brach & Fraser). In this view, cultural competency goes beyond cultural awareness or even sensitivity. Indeed, it includes not only the possession of cultural knowledge and respect for differing cultural perspectives, but also having skills and being able to use them effectively in cross-cultural settings. It also carries the connotation of an ongoing commitment or institutionalization of appropriate practices and policies for diverse populations (Brach & Fraser). While the field is still relatively young, culturally competent strategies and techniques usually include items in one or more of the following categories. (1) Interpreter services are the most commonly envisioned cultural competence enhancement strategy (Brach & Fraser; Smedley et al.). Providing such services is indeed one of the most obvious ways to improve communication and enhance understanding in the healthcare environment. (2) Recruitment and retention of minority staff is considered an important part of cultural competency (Brach & Fraser; Smedley et al.). Minority staff possess shared cultural experiences and beliefs with minority patients and as such may be able to more effectively communicate with other minority patients. (3) Utilization of specific cultural competence training programs is another element of culturally competent healthcare systems. Cultural proficiency does not just happen. Rather, specific knowledge and certain skills can be taught that may improve doctor–patient interactions. (4) Employing and valuing the efforts of natural lay leaders such as community health workers (CHW) have been deemed another key determinant of cultural competency (Brach & Fraser). All of the world's cultures have a lay healthcare system, comprising natural helpers or community members to whom neighbors can turn for social encouragement and assistance (Satterfield, Burd, Valez, Hosey, & Shield, 2002). The origins of the development of a CHW workforce may in part be traced to the work of seventeenth century Russian Feldshers. Feldshers were lay citizens who underwent a year-long training program in preparation to care for Russian civilian and military populations (Gibbons, 2006). Later, the same model was seen in the work of the Chinese "barefoot doctor" program (Gibbons) and in the Village Health Worker model of the World Health Organization (Bender & Pitkin, 1987). Today, approximately 1,400 community health representatives work with programs in over 560 federally recognized American-Indian and Alaska Native people (Gibbons).

In the scientific literature, CHWs have been referred to by more than 30 different names, including lay health advisors, health aides, promatoras, consejeras, dumas, and patient navigators. Patient navigators comprise a subset of CHWs whose care coordination activities focus on the clinical encounter and do not generally focus on patient outreach, case findings, primary prevention, or posttherapeutic case management (Gibbons, 2006). While patient navigator activities may indeed occur in the community, they are primarily designed to facilitate timely and appropriate utilization of the healthcare system.

There are several generally recognized reasons why the patient navigator approach is promising. First, few of the millions of dollars that are spent on low-income communities each year fund employment for residents of those communities (Gibbons, 2006). Secondly, indigenous workers are better able to reach and communicate with community residents and thereby provide culturally appropriate outreach and cultural linkages between communities and delivery systems. Because they are better equipped to provide culturally appropriate services, well-designed and implemented CHW programs may reduce costs by providing health education screening, detection, and basic emergency care. They may also improve quality by contributing to patient–provider communication, continuity of care, and consumer protection (Witmer, Seifer, Finocchio, Leslie, & O'Neil, 1995).

(5) Inclusion and respect of the values and perspectives of family and community members (Brach & Fraser, 2000) is another quality found among culturally competent providers and healthcare systems. In the US, patient autonomy has become a principle of paramount importance. However, other cultures of the world may value family and community perspectives when making important health and

healthcare decisions (Brach & Fraser). Involving these individuals may be essential in obtaining consent and maintaining adherence to treatment regimens (Brach & Fraser). (6) Making specific administrative and organizational accommodations, another cultural competency strategy, may provide evidence of true commitment to the promotion of the well-being of all patients (Brach & Fraser). A variety of strategies are envisioned here which may range from clinic locations and nonstandard hours of operation to the utilization of mobile units and facilities that can better access minority community members (Brach & Fraser). Finally, some cultural competency advocates encourage a total emersion into the local indigenous culture (Brach & Fraser). Once accomplished, this has been reported to facilitate significant enhancements in awareness, sensitivity, and specific skills needed for effective cross-cultural working relationships (Brach & Fraser).

There are several potential mechanisms through which these cultural competency strategies may work to reduce racial and ethnic disparities in health care. These include facilitating more successful patient education, changing patient healthcare-seeking behaviors or healthcare preferences, facilitating more appropriate testing and screening and as such fewer missed opportunities for detection and treatment (Brach & Fraser, 2000). Cultural competence may also help providers learn of any complimentary or alternative therapies being used by patients (Brach & Fraser). This would help physicians avoid dangerous errors or drug interactions that may occur between prescribed medications and other substances of which the clinician may not be aware. Culturally competent systems may facilitate greater long-term adherence to therapy and follow-up care. Finally, culturally competent systems facilitate patient choice by expanding minority patients' pool of high-quality providers on whom they can rely for their healthcare needs (Brach & Fraser).

Summary

The fragmentary nature of the US healthcare system may significantly contribute to the development and persistence of healthcare disparities by inhibiting the continuity and cohesiveness of care provided to patients. Multiple health plan coverage options, institutionally imposed physician cost constraints, and differential geographic availability of needed healthcare services all likely contribute to problems which may result in fragmented healthcare delivery. Increasingly, limited diversity among healthcare professionals and the lack of culturally competent healthcare systems are also being seen as contributors to healthcare disparities.

References

Anderson, L., Scrimshaw, S., Fullilove, M., Fielding, J., & Normand, J. (2003). Culturally competent healthcare systems: A systematic review. *American Journal of Preventive Medicine, 24*, 68–79.

Baicker, K., Chandra, A., & Skinner, J. S. (2005). Geographic variation in health care and the problem of measuring racial disparities. *Perspectives in Biology and Medicine, 48,* S42–S53.

Baicker, K., Chandra, A., Skinner, J. S., & Wennberg, J. E. (2004). Who you are and where you live: How race and geography affect the treatment of medicare beneficiaries. *Health Affairs (Project Hope), (Suppl Web Exclusive),* VAR33–VAR44.

Bender, D. E., & Pitkin, K. (1987). Bridging the gap: The village health worker as the cornerstone of the primary health care model. *Social Science & Medicine, 24,* 515–528.

Betancourt, J., Green, A., & Carrillo, E. (2002). *Cultural competence in healthcare: Emerging frameworks and practical approaches* (Rep. No. 576). Washington, DC: The Commonwealth Fund.

Betancourt, J. R., & Maina, A. W. (2004). The Institute of Medicine report "Unequal Treatment": Implications for academic health centers. The *Mount Sinai Journal of .Medicine, 71,* 314–321.

Blustein, J., & Weitzman, B. C. (1995). Access to hospitals with high-technology cardiac services: How is race important? *American Journal of Public Health, 85,* 345–351.

Brach, C., & Fraser, I. (2000). Can cultural competency reduce racila and ethnic disparities? A review and conceptual model. *Medical Care Research and Review, 57,* 181–217.

Brennan, T. A., Hebert, L. E., Laird, N. M., Lawthers, A., Thorpe, K. E., Leape, L. L., et al. (1991). Hospital characteristics associated with adverse events and substandard care. *JAMA: The Journal of the American Medical Association, 265,* 3265–3269.

Brennan, T. A., Leape, L. L., Laird, N. M., Hebert, L., Localio, A. R., Lawthers, A. G., et al. (1991). Incidence of adverse events and negligence in hospitalized patients. Results of the Harvard Medical Practice Study I. *The New England Journal of Medicine, 324,* 370–376.

Brennan, T. A., Leape, L. L., Laird, N. M., Localio, A. R., & Hiatt, H. H. (1990). Incidence of adverse events and negligent care in hospitalized patients. *Transactions of the Association of American Physicians, 103,* 137–144.

Cone, D. C., Richardson, L. D., Todd, K. H., Betancourt, J. R., & Lowe, R. A. (2003). Health care disparities in emergency medicine. *Academic Emergency Medicine, 10,* 1176–1183.

Cooper-Patrick, L., Gallo, J. J., Gonzales, J. J., Vu, H. T., Powe, N. R., Nelson, C., et al. (1999). Race, gender, and partnership in the patient–physician relationship. *JAMA: The Journal of the American Medical Association, 282,* 583–589.

Fulcher, C. L., & Kaukinen, C. E. (2004). Visualizing the infrastructure of US healthcare using Internet GIS: A community health informatics approach for reducing health disparities. *Medinfo, 11,* 1197–1201.

Fulcher, C., & Kaukinen, C. (2005). Mapping and visualizing the location HIV service providers: An exploratory spatial analysis of Toronto neighborhoods. *AIDS Care, 17,* 386–396.

Gibbons, M. C. (2006). Common ground: Exploring policy approaches to addressing racial disparities from the left and the right. *The Journal of Healthcare Law and Policy, 9,* 48–76.

Gray, B., & Stoddard, J. J. (1997). Patient–physician pairing: Does racial and ethnic congruity influence selection of a regular physician? *Journal of Community Health, 22,* 247–259.

IOM Committee on Quality of Healthcare in America. (2001). *Crossing the quality chasm: A new health system for the 21st century.* Washington, DC: National Academy Press.

Kaplan, S. H., Gandek, B., Greenfield, S., Rogers, W., & Ware, J. E. (1995). Patient and visit characteristics related to physicians' participatory decision-making style. Results from the Medical Outcomes Study. *Medical Care, 33,* 1176–1187.

Kaukinen, C., & Fulcher, C. (2006). Mapping the social demography and location of HIV services across Toronto neighbourhoods. *Health & Social Care in the Community, 14,* 37–48.

Keith, S. N., Bell, R. M., Swanson, A. G., & Williams, A. P. (1985). Effects of affirmative action in medical schools. A study of the class of 1975. *The New England Journal of Medicine, 313,* 1519–1525.

Kennedy, E. M. (2005). The role of the federal government in eliminating health disparities. *Health Affairs (Project Hope), 24,* 452–458.

Kohn, L., Corrigan, J., & Donaldson, M. (2000). *To err is human: Building a safer health system*. Washington, DC: National Academy Press.

Komaromy, M., Grumbach, K., Drake, M., Vranizan, K., Lurie, N., Keane, D., et al. (1996). The role of black and Hispanic physicians in providing health care for underserved populations. *The New England Journal of Medicine, 334*, 1305–1310.

Kurth, T., Kase, C. S., Berger, K., Schaeffner, E. S., Buring, J. E., & Gaziano, J. M. (2003). Smoking and the risk of hemorrhagic stroke in men. *Stroke, 34*, 1151–1155.

Leape, L. L., Brennan, T. A., Laird, N., Lawthers, A. G., Localio, A. R., Barnes, B. A., et al. (1991). The nature of adverse events in hospitalized patients. Results of the Harvard Medical Practice Study II. *The New England Journal of Medicine, 324*, 377–384.

Leape, L. L., Hilborne, L. H., Bell, R., Kamberg, C., & Brook, R. H. (1999). Under use of cardiac procedures: Do women, ethnic minorities, and the uninsured fail to receive needed revascularization? *Annals of Internal Medicine, 130*, 183–192.

Lloyd, S. M., Jr., Johnson, D. G., & Mann, M. (1978). Survey of graduates of a traditionally black college of medicine. *Journal of Medical Education, 53*, 640–650.

McPherson, K., Wennberg, J. E., Hovind, O. B., & Clifford, P. (1982). Small-area variations in the use of common surgical procedures: An international comparison of New England, England, and Norway. *The New England Journal of Medicine, 307*, 1310–1314.

Morrison, R. S., Wallenstein, S., Natale, D. K., Senzel, R. S., & Huang, L. L. (2000). "We don't carry that" – Failure of pharmacies in predominantly nonwhite neighborhoods to stock opioid analgesics. *The New England Journal of Medicine, 342*, 1023–1026.

Palepu, A., Carr, P. L., Friedman, R. H., Amos, H., Ash, A. S., & Moskowitz, M. A. (1998). Minority faculty and academic rank in medicine. *JAMA: The Journal of the American Medical Association, 280*, 767–771.

Phibbs, C. S., & Luft, H. S. (1995). Correlation of travel time on roads versus straight line distance. *Medical Care Research and Review, 52*, 532–542.

Satterfield, D., Burd, C., Valez, L., Hosey, G., & Shield, J. (2002). The "in-between people": Participation of CHR's in diabetes prevention and care in American Indian and Alaska native communities. *Health Promotion Practice, 3*, 166–175.

Schneider, E. C., Zaslavsky, A. M., & Epstein, A. M. (2002). Racial disparities in the quality of care for enrollees in medicare managed care. *JAMA: The Journal of the American Medical Association, 287*, 1288–1294.

Smedley, B. D., Stith, A. Y., & Nelson, A. R. (2003). *Unequal treatment: Confronting racial and ethnic disparities in healthcare*. Washington, DC: National Academy Press.

Susi, L., & Mascarenhas, A. K. (2002). Using a geographical information system to map the distribution of dentists in Ohio. *Journal of the American Dental Association, 133*, 636–642.

Vanasse, A., Niyonsenga, T., Courteau, J., Gregoire, J. P., Hemiari, A., Loslier, J., et al. (2005). Spatial variation in the management and outcomes of acute coronary syndrome. *BMC Cardiovascular Disorders, 5*, 21.

Vining, B. A., Lurie, N., & Huang, Z. (2003). Racial variation in quality of care among Medicare + choice enrollees. *Health Affairs (Project Hope), 21*, 224–230.

Witmer, A., Seifer, S. D., Finocchio, L., Leslie, J., & O'Neil, E. H. (1995). Community health workers: Integral members of the health care work force. *American Journal of Public Health, 85*, 1055–1058.

Zipes, D. P., Libby, P., Bonow, R. O., & Braunwald, E. (Eds.). (2005). *Braunwald's heart disease* (7th ed.). Philadelphia: Elsevier-Saunders.

5
The Social "Nonmedical" Determinants of Health

Nadra Tyus and Michael Christopher Gibbons

Contemporary and Future Healthcare Dynamics

Over the past decade, a rapidly expanding body of scientific evidence has documented differences in health status among US racial and ethnic groups. These disparities in health status are generally thought to be related to factors beyond the scope of the healthcare system (Smedley, Stith, & Nelson, 2003). In contrast, disparities in health care are thought to be limited to determinants more closely related to the healthcare system. Obviously, the logic of such reasoning is clear. However, mounting evidence suggests that as a practical matter, this distinction may be of little value. This is in part because growing proportions of the population are living with chronic diseases. Approximately 60% of UK citizens and 50% of US citizens report having at least one chronic disease. These numbers are expected to rise further in the near future. Additionally, both US and European healthcare systems are oriented toward acute episodic inpatient treatment, and, as such, have only limited ability in their current configurations to respond adequately to this growing problem. Indeed, the World Health Organization (WHO) has suggested that healthcare systems worldwide are struggling to meet the needs of population's suffering from chronic diseases (National Health Service, 2004). Obviously then, fragmented healthcare delivery systems and increasing numbers of individuals with multiple comorbid conditions contribute directly to poor quality care, unnecessary medical errors, and poor patient outcomes (IOM Committee on Quality of Healthcare in America, 2001; National Health Service), thus also contributing to healthcare disparities.

Effective chronic care, unlike acute treatment care, is a much more collaborative process between patients and providers. It involves a much larger reliance on provider directed self-care, community-based health risk management, disease management, care coordination, and care facilitation. Over time, this community-based care model will be increasingly provided by nonphysician healthcare professionals such as family members, friends, and associates (IOM Committee on Quality of Healthcare in America, 2001; National Health Service, 2004). Given this reality, medical care systems of the future will need to develop a robust population perspective in addition to the more traditional medical model of individualized medicine. Historically, the population perspective has largely occupied the domain of Public Health while individualized health issues belonged to medical care (2001). In the past, this distinction may have been useful and practical. However, a shift away from only individualized acute hospital based care to care that predominantly occurs in communities and a growing realization of the importance of neighborhood and community factors on health care outcomes suggest a diminished value of this dichotomization.

Another development mitigating against the utility of a dichotomization of "medical factors" and "health factors" in clinical medicine is the need for a greater focus on prevention and behavioral factors in the US healthcare system (Singer & Ryff, 2001). Ultimately, sustaining health, recovering from disease, or achieving optimal clinical results will usually require some form of behavior change. This may range from stress reduction to increased physical activity, medication adherence, and timely follow-up visits. Evidence from the behavioral sciences strongly suggests that to achieve these behavioral goals, information alone is insufficient, particularly over a long period of time (Carleton, Lasater, Assaf, Feldman, & McKinlay, 1995; Farquhar et al., 1990; *Health Education and Health Behavior: Theory, Research and Practice* 1997; Luepker et al., 1994). Yet, many medical professionals advocate health educational interventions as a primary means of achieving patient behavior change.

Behavioral science knowledge can also aid the understanding and addressing of healthcare disparities. For example, among African-Americans, various sociocultural factors are being recognized as important contributors to disparities in obesity, hypertension, and diabetes rates (Watkins, 2004). The belief that health outcomes are ordained by God and therefore cannot be changed, also referred to as fatalism, has been documented as a cultural factor contributing to healthcare outcomes among African-Americans (Kressin & Petersen, 2001). It has even been noted that similar culturally determined attitudes and beliefs (myths) may impact decision making among African-American patients and contribute to hypertensive inequalities (Ferguson et al., 1998). For instance, it has been documented that African-American men incorrectly described as being healthy and symptom free and as a result, self-adjusted their medication usage depending on the existence of "symptoms." In addition, these men considered buying antihypertensive medications a luxury, because of their high cost. They also think that seeking help for hypertension is a sign of weakness or laziness (Rose, Kim, Dennison, & Hill, 2000). These attitudes and beliefs may, in part, be responsible for the findings of suboptimal medication adherence and inadequate self-monitoring of blood pressure among African-Americans (Chobanian et al., 2003). Finally, evidence indicates as many as 50% of newly diagnosed hypertensives discontinue use of prescribed medications within 1 year of diagnosis and up to 50% of the remaining patients do not take their medications as prescribed (Friday, 1999). Issues of poor medication adherence and inadequate self-monitoring of blood pressure are problems in the entire hypertensive population and are especially problematic among African-American patients in the US (Artinian, Washington, & Templin, 2001; Friday; Hill et al., 1999; Rose et al.).

Disparities in Health Status

The earliest reported observation of a hypothesized association between socioenvironmental risk factors and health status occurred in Italy over three centuries ago
when Bernardino Ramazzini detailed an unusually high frequency of breast cancer
in Catholic nuns (Wilson, Jones, Coussens, & Hanna, 2002). Not long thereafter in
1775, British surgeon Sir Percival Pott reported a cluster of scrotal cancer cases
among British chimney sweeps (Wilson et al.). By the mid-nineteenth century,
large-scale epidemiologic evidence began to corroborate these early observations.
In 1840, Edwin Chadwick, a British civil servant and statistician, demonstrated
mortality differentials between the social classes living in Liverpool, England.
Chadwick asserted that these differences were likely due to poverty and lifestyle
factors common to the poorer working classes (Macintyre, 1997). German physician Rudolph Virchow went a step further when, in 1849, he asserted that because
diseases of the populace are traceable to defects in society, the focus of medicine
should shift from changing the individual to that of changing the society (Amick,
Levine, Tarlov, & Walsh, 1995). Finally, in France, French physician Louis
Villerme recommended improving school and working conditions as social interventions that would reduce class differences in mortality (Amick et al.). Thus, in
Europe, by the beginning of the twentieth century, the existence of class variations
in morbidity and mortality was clearly evident in the scientific literature
(Macintyre).

Throughout the twentieth century the study of social class differences in health
status continued across Europe, especially in Britain where epidemiologists began
using decennial census data to evaluate national mortality trends. The insights gained
from these analyses enabled them to construct an occupational social class grading
system that correlated inversely with infant mortality. It also was the basis of the
claim made by the Registrar General of Britain that at least 40% of British infant
mortality was entirely preventable if the social conditions of poor infants could be
elevated to that of upper-class infants (Macintyre, 1997).

Two British researchers, Titmuss and Logan, evaluated regional class-based
mortality trends and documented that the disparity in infant mortality rates between
upper- and lower-class infants continued to increase from 1910 to 1950 (Macintyre,
1997). This data, along with the Depression and World War II, encouraged the
British government in 1942, to respond by instituting the welfare state and promoting several policy initiatives designed to address the "five giants of Want, Disease,
Ignorance, Squalor, and Idleness" (Macintyre; Acheson, 1998). Despite this government investment, however, problems attributable to social inequalities and
inadequate access to health care persisted. In fact, by the mid 1970s, some 30 years
later, the evidence seemed to indicate that the problems were still increasing and
that the health of British citizens was slipping behind that of other industrialized
nations (Acheson). Thus, in 1977, the British government formed the Research
Working Group on Inequalities in Health and selected Sir Douglas Black as its
chair. The committee's report, issued three years later in 1980, became known as

the Black Report, and it represents the first attempt by a national government to systematically study, understand, and explain health inequalities (Acheson). In summary, the health improvement recommendations of the report emphasized the need to improve the physical and the social environment in which the poor and lower classes lived (Acheson).

Domestic Recognition of Disparities in Health Status

In 1984, the US Department of Health and Human Services released a report on the health of the nation, entitled *"Health, United States, 1983"* (NCHS, 1983). The report documented that, while the overall health of the nation showed significant progress, major disparities existed in "the burden of death and illness experienced by Blacks and other minority Americans as compared with the nation's population as a whole" (NCHS). In response to the disparities identified in the report, the secretary of the Department of Health and Human Services established a task force on Black and minority health – the first time that the US government formed a group of experts to conduct a comprehensive study of minority health problems. In 1985, release of the "Report of the Secretary's Task Force on Black and Minority Health" significantly raised awareness of the disparate health of the country's minority groups as compared to the White majority population (Mayberry, Mili, & Ofili, 2000).

While minorities are more likely than Whites to be of low SES, researchers also identified disparities among the well educated and employed (Marmot, Rose, Shipley, & Hamilton, 1978). This realization led researchers to suggest that certain community and societal level factors, including stress (Marmot, 1986; Sapolsky & Mott, 1987), early life experiences (Tager, Weiss, Munoz, Rosner, & Speizer, 1983), social support (Berkman & Kawachi, 2000), food availability (Marmot & Wilkinson, 2006), and neighborhood and community factors (Amick et al., 1995) were important nonmedical or social determinants of health status (Amick et al.; Brennan, Leape, Laird, Localio, & Hiatt, 1990; Wilkinson, 1996).

Social Determinants of Health

Stress and Health

Stress has short-term and long-term effects on the body. Given the right balance of factors the effect is positive. It is beginning to be realized that social and psychological circumstances may damage health over the long term (Marmot & Wilkinson, 2006; Wilkinson, 1996). Chronic anxiety, insecurity, and social isolation appear to undermine health (Marmot & Wilkinson). The ability of psychological factors like stress to affect health is biologically plausible (Berkman & Kawachi, 2000). The excessive or prolonged activation of biologic stress responses within the body may enhance the risk of depression, diabetes, high blood pressure, heart attack, and increase disease susceptibility (Marmot & Wilkinson). The poor and minorities are at increased risk for many of these health problems. The clustering and accumulation of psychological disadvantage, perhaps beginning as early as childhood, is being investigated as a potential contributor to these disparities (Marmot, 1986; Marmot, Ryff, Bumpass, Shipley, & Marks, 1997; Marmot & Wilkinson).

Early Life Experiences

Social experiences can exert a significant effect on health from in utero development of the fetus through infancy and childhood. The concept of biological programming is founded on the notion that at discrete points early in embryological development of the fetus unique periods of time exist, in which an insult, could exert detrimental effects at some point later in the process of growth and development (Marmot & Wilkinson, 2006). Poor adult health consequences have been associated with poor growth in early life. These include blood pressure, cardiovascular disease, diabetes (Cheung, Low, Osmond, Barker, & Karlberg, 2000; Miura et al., 2001; Smith et al., 2001), and breast cancer (De Stavola et al., 2004). Social factors that affect early life growth and development include maternal smoking or alcohol consumption, poor maternal diet, or illicit drug use.

Social Support

Emile Durkheim, a French sociologist in the late nineteenth century was one of the first to propose that social factors could influence health (Berkman & Kawachi, 2000). In his classic work *Le Suicide*, Durkheim noted that suicide had to be one of the most individualized acts possible. As such, the occurrence of suicide should be largely random in a large population. Yet, his work demonstrated for the first time that suicide rates in Europe were not random and thus had to be influenced by some other factor present in the larger society (Berkman & Kawachi). Upon further investigation Durkheim found that suicide rates varied inversely with the degree of social integration experienced by an individual (Berkman & Kawachi). Several years later American psychiatrist John Bowlby proposed his attachment theory in which he describes the need for close human relationships among children and adults (Berkman & Kawachi). He proposed that these attachments provided psychological protection which forms the basis for marital relationships in adulthood (Berkman & Kawachi). By the 1950s, anthropologists and sociologists began looking at the structure and dynamics of the relationships people were engaged in as a means of understanding human behavior. Finally by the mid 1970s, epidemiologists began suggesting a link between social support or social relationships and disease risk. Over the next two decades, several studies demonstrated that the lack of social support was consistently associated with higher mortality risk from almost every cause of death (Berkman & Kawachi). Since then scientists have studied both qualitative and quantitative aspects of social relationship. While there is some level of imprecision in the definitions and measures used, in general the weight of the scientific evidence seems to support the notion that greater amounts of social connectedness, no matter how it is measured, is associated with health benefits (Berkman & Kawachi).

Food Availability

A good diet and adequate food supply are central for promoting health and well-being. A shortage of food and lack of variety increase the risk of poor health. On the other hand excessive intake of certain foods contributes to cardiovascular diseases, diabetes, cancer, degenerative eye diseases, obesity, and dental caries (Marmot & Wilkinson, 2006). The important public health issue is the availability and cost of healthy, nutritious food. Access to good, affordable food makes more difference to what people eat than health education (Marmot & Wilkinson). Several studies have documented that the types of food and grocery store establishments differ in White vs. minority communities. In general the White communities have the larger national chain grocery stores while the minority communities tend to have the small corner food stores with much more limited selection of foods, particularly fresh fruits and vegetables (Moore & Diez Roux, 2006; Morland, Wing, Diez, & Poole, 2002). In addition it has been shown that the cost of food differs by as much as 30% between these types of food stores. The higher costs tend to be found in the minority grocery stores where the patrons have lower financial resources at baseline (Diez Roux, 2001; Moore & Diez Roux; Morland et al.). In the case of liquor establishments, store location and number of stores in a given community were shown to be associated with amount of alcohol ingested per capita in the local community and associated with dietary nutrient intake by local community residents (LaVeist & Wallace, 2000). These stores are often disproportionately located in minority neighborhoods.

Community and Neighborhood

The physical environmental characteristics exert important effects on communities and the health of its population (Amick et al., 1995). The most important factors include air, water pollution, geographic location (urban vs. rural), noise level, housing and transportation issues. The quality of a community's air and water resources are among the most visible aspects of the physical environment (Amick et al.).

Environmental, behavioral, and occupational exposures to well-known pulmonary carcinogens, including tobacco, asbestos, radon, polycyclic aromatic hydrocarbons (PAHs), and heterocyclic amines are well documented (Alberg & Samet, 2003; Franceschi & Bidoli, 1999; Pitot, 2002). Individuals living in housing units located close to a factory spewing carcinogenic emissions from its smoke stack might be expected to experience higher carcinogenic exposure levels over time compared to ambient air exposures in individuals who live in rural areas. In fact, location of urban residence has been associated with increased personal exposure and an increased lifetime risk of cancer (Kinney, Chillrud, Ramstrom, Ross, & Stansfeld, 2002; Morello-Frosch, Pastor, Porras, & Sadd, 2002). In addition, carcinogenic exposures from other sources like diesel exhaust fumes may be significantly higher in urban communities than exposures to these same carcinogens in rural environments.

Summary

While in the past a distinction between healthcare disparities and health disparities has been made, increasingly as our healthcare system moves toward more, patient-centered, community-based, chronic disease care, the distinctions will become less relevant. This is because the distinction between health care and social care will become blurred. Issues of behavior and sociocultural issues formerly considered less relevant to healthcare, are assuming new relevance. As such medical researchers have begun to more closely examine the so-called social determinants of health and their relationship to healthcare and health outcomes.

References

Acheson, D. (1998). *Independent inquiry into inequalities in health*. London: The Stationery Office.
Alberg, A. J., & Samet, J. M. (2003). Epidemiology of lung cancer. *Chest, 123*, 21S–49S.
Amick, B. C., Levine, S., Tarlov, A. R., & Walsh, D. C. (1995). *Society and health*. New York: Oxford University Press.
Artinian, N. T., Washington, O. G., & Templin, T. N. (2001). Effects of home telemonitoring and community-based monitoring on blood pressure control in urban African Americans: A pilot study. *Heart Lung, 30*, 191–199.
Berkman, L. F., & Kawachi, I. (2000). *Social epidemiology*. New York: Oxford University Press.
Brennan, T. A., Leape, L. L., Laird, N. M., Localio, A. R., & Hiatt, H. H. (1990). Incidence of adverse events and negligent care in hospitalized patients. *Transactions of the Association of American Physicians, 103*, 137–144.
Carleton, R. A., Lasater, T. M., Assaf, A. R., Feldman, H. A., & McKinlay, S. (1995). The Pawtucket Heart Health Program: Community changes in cardiovascular risk factors and projected disease risk. *American Journal of Public Health, 85*, 777–785.

Cheung, Y. B., Low, L., Osmond, C., Barker, D., & Karlberg, J. (2000). Fetal growth and early postnatal growth are related to blood pressure in adults. *Hypertension, 36*, 795–800.

Chobanian, A. V., Bakris, G. L., Black, H. R., Cushman, W. C., Green, L. A., Izzo, J. L., Jr., et al. (2003). The seventh report of the joint national committee on prevention, detection, evaluation, and treatment of high blood pressure: The JNC 7 report. *JAMA: The Journal of the American Medical Association, 289*, 2560–2572.

De Stavola, B. L., dos, S. S. I., McCormack, V., Hardy, R. J., Kuh, D. J., & Wadsworth, M. E. (2004). Childhood growth and breast cancer. *American Journal of Epidemiology, 159*, 671–682.

Diez Roux, A. V. (2001). Investigating neighborhood and area effects on health. *American Journal of Public Health, 91*, 1783–1789.

Farquhar, J. W., Fortmann, S. P., Flora, J. A., Taylor, C. B., Haskell, W. L., Williams, P. T., et al. (1990). Effects of communitywide education on cardiovascular disease risk factors. The Stanford Five-City Project. *JAMA: The Journal of the American Medical Association, 264*, 359–365.

Ferguson, J. A., Weinberger, M., Westmoreland, G. R., Mamlin, L. A., Segar, D. S., Greene, J. Y., et al. (1998). Racial disparity in cardiac decision making: Results from patient focus groups. *Archives of Internal Medicine, 158*, 1450–1453.

Franceschi, S., & Bidoli, E. (1999). The epidemiology of lung cancer. *Annals of Oncology, 10*(Suppl. 5), S3–S6.

Friday, G. H. (1999). Antihypertensive medication compliance in African-American stroke patients: Behavioral epidemiology and interventions. *Neuroepidemiology, 18*, 223–230.

Health education and health behavior: Theory, research and practice (2nd ed.). (1997). San Francisco, CA: Jose-Bass.

Hill, M., Bone, L., Kim, M., Miller, D., Dennison, C., & Levine, D. (1999). Barriers to hypertension care and control in young urban black men. *American Journal of Hypertension, 12*, 951–958.

IOM Committee on Quality of Healthcare in America. (2001). *Crossing the quality chasm: A new health system for the 21st century*. Washington, DC: National Academy Press.

Kinney, P., Chillrud, S., Ramstrom, S., Ross, J., & Stansfeld, S. A. (2002). Exposure to multiple air toxics in New York city. *Environmental Health Perspectives, 110*(Suppl. 4), 539–546.

Kressin, N. R., & Petersen, L. A. (2001). Racial differences in the use of invasive cardiovascular procedures: Review of the literature and prescription for future research. *Annals of Internal Medicine, 135*, 352–366.

LaVeist, T. A., & Wallace, J. M., Jr. (2000). Health risk and inequitable distribution of liquor stores in African American neighborhood. *Social Science & Medicine, 51*, 613–617.

Luepker, R. V., Murray, D. M., Jacobs, D. R., Jr., Mittelmark, M. B., Bracht, N., Carlaw, R., et al. (1994). Community education for cardiovascular disease prevention: Risk factor changes in the Minnesota Heart Health Program. *American Journal of Public Health, 84*, 1383–1393.

Macintyre, S. (1997). The Black report and beyond: What are the issues? *Social Science & Medcine, 44*, 723–745.

Marmot, M. G. (1986). Does stress cause heart attacks? *Postgraduate Medical Journal, 62*, 683–686.

Marmot, M. G., Rose, G., Shipley, M., & Hamilton, P. J. (1978). Employment grade and coronary heart disease in British civil servants. *Journal of Epidemiology and Community Health, 32*, 244–249.

Marmot, M., Ryff, C. D., Bumpass, L. L., Shipley, M., & Marks, N. F. (1997). Social inequalities in health: Next questions and converging evidence. *Social Science & Medicine, 44*, 901–910.

Marmot, M., & Wilkinson, R. G. (2006). *Social determinants of health*. (2nd ed.). Oxford: Oxford University Press.

Mayberry, R. M., Mili, F., & Ofili, E. (2000). Racial and ethnic differences in access to medical care. *Medical Care Research and Review, 57*(Suppl. 1), 108–145.

Medical Informatics (2nd ed.). (2001). New York, NY: Springer.

Miura, K., Nakagawa, H., Tabata, M., Morikawa, Y., Nishijo, M., & Kagamimori, S. (2001). Birth weight, childhood growth, and cardiovascular disease risk factors in Japanese aged 20 years. *American Journal of Epidemiology, 153*, 783–789.

Moore, L., & Diez Roux, A. (2006). Associations of neighborhood characteristics with the location and type of food stores. *American Journal of Public Health, 96*, 325–331.

Morello-Frosch, R., Pastor, M., Porras, C., & Sadd, J. (2002). Environmental justice and regional inequality in southern California: Implications for future research. *Environmental Health Perspectives, 110*(Suppl. 2), 149–154.

Morland, K., Wing, S., Diez, R. A., & Poole, C. (2002). Neighborhood characteristics associated with the location of food stores and food service places. *American Journal of Preventive Medicine, 22*, 23–29.

National Health Service. (2004). *Chronic disease management: A compendium of information*. London, England: UK Department of Health.

NCHS. (1983). *NCHS: Health, United States, 1983; and prevention profile* (Rep. No. (PHS) 84–1232). Washington, DC: US Government Printing Office.

Pitot, H. C. (2002). The host–tumor relationship. In H. C. Pitot (Ed.), *Fundamentals of oncology* (4 ed., pp. 743–781). New York: Marcel Dekker, Inc.

Rose, L., Kim, M., Dennison, C., & Hill, M. (2000). The context of adherence for African-Americans with high blood pressure. *Journal of Advanced Nursing, 32*, 587–594.

Sapolsky, R. M., & Mott, G. E. (1987). Social subordinance in wild baboons is associated with suppressed high density lipoprotein–cholesterol concentrations: The possible role of chronic social stress. *Endocrinology, 121*, 1605–1610.

Singer, B. H., & Ryff, C. D. (2001). *New horizons in health: An integrative approach*. Washington, DC: National Academy Press.

Smedley, B. D., Stith, A. Y., & Nelson, A. R. (2003). *Unequal treatment; Confronting racial and ethnic disparities in healthcare*. Washington, DC: National Academy Press.

Smith, G. D., Greenwood, R., Gunnell, D., Sweetnam, P., Yarnell, J., & Elwood, P. (2001). Leg length, insulin resistance, and coronary heart disease risk: The Caerphilly Study. *Journal of Epidemiology and Community Health, 55*, 867–872.

Tager, I. B., Weiss, S. T., Munoz, A., Rosner, B., & Speizer, F. E. (1983). Longitudinal study of the effects of maternal smoking on pulmonary function in children. *The New England Journal of Medicine, 309*, 699–703.

Watkins, L. O. (2004). Perspectives on coronary heart disease in African Americans. *Reviews in Cardiovascular Medicine, 5*(Suppl. 3), S3–S13.

Wilkinson, R. G. (1996). *Unhealthy societies: The afflictions of inequalities*. New York: Routledge.

Wilson, S., Jones, L., Coussens, C., & Hanna, K. (2002). *Cancer and the environment; Gene–environment interaction*. Washington, DC: National Academy Press.

Section II

6
The Role of the Internet in American Life

Michael Christopher Gibbons

It is not possible to consider current and future opportunities for health care in the computer and information technologies without considering the role of the Internet in American life. While the rise of the Internet in society provided the foundation for the increasing role of the Internet in health and health care, there is growing realization that the growing role of the Internet in health and health care is not only changing the nature of health care, but also, in several ways, fundamentally changing the way we live in society. Undoubtedly, these societal changes will have significant implications for the personalized, community-based healthcare system of the future. Because of the pervasiveness of the impact of the Internet and because these changes are and will continue to impact health and health care, this chapter will briefly discuss the role of the Internet in society today.

The Rise of the Internet in Society

If there is a time that could be considered the dawn of the modern Internet, it was probably on October 13, 1994 when Netscape's Mosaic browser was made available free on a company Web site (Rainie et al., 2005). On a single day, thousands of people began experiencing the World-Wide Web in a whole new way (Rainie et al.). Thirteen years later, the Internet has reached into just about every important facet of modern life (Rainie et al.).

Internet Penetration

In 1995, just 15% of individuals were using the Internet. They were doing so primarily via Bulletin Board Services or proprietary businesses like CompuServe and Prodigy. Today, Internet use continues to soar with 147 million Americans (73%) being Internet users (Madden, 2007). In the last year alone there has been a 7% (14 million people) increase in Internet usage in the US (Madden). Many Americans believe that the Internet has helped them improve their lives (Madden). For example, 32% of

Americans say that the Internet has greatly improved their shopping, 33% of Americans say that the Internet has greatly improved the way they pursue hobbies and interests, 35% say the Internet has greatly improved their ability to do their jobs, and 20% of Americans indicate that the Internet has greatly improved the way they get information about health care (Madden). It appears that as utilization of the Internet grows, so does familiarity and perceived level of benefit. Daily Internet users are twice as likely as occasional users to indicate that the Internet has improved their ability to do their job "a lot" (Madden).

The growth in Internet use has not been uniform across the country. The highest rates (approx 70%) are seen along the Atlantic and Pacific coasts (Spooner, 2003). Relatively high rates (approx 60%) are seen in the Rocky mountain and Border States, while moderately low rates (approx 55%) are seen in the southeastern and Industrial Midwest states (Spooner). The lowest rates in the US (<50%) are seen in the south (Spooner). This regional variation in Internet use is related to education and income levels (Spooner). In general, those regions that have more people with substantial household incomes and college degrees tend to have a higher proportion of Internet users. California, the National Capital region, and New England have large populations of wealthy, highly educated people. As such, these regions are among the most highly wired in the US. On the other hand, the South has the lowest household income and education levels among its overall population compared to other regions and likewise it has the lowest level of Internet penetration among adults (Spooner).

In terms of online activities, Midwesterners are very much interested in getting their news online while users in the Mountain States are not avid online news users. Compared with other regions, a high proportion of those in the South look for health information online. Those using the Web on the west coast are the least likely to spend time simply browsing the Internet for fun. However, in terms of shopping, users in New England and California are most likely to shop online. Individuals online in the South and Southeast are the least likely to engage in online shopping (Spooner, 2003).

Interestingly, it is possible to construct fairly detailed online regional user profiles. For example, users in New England tend to be wealthier and educated. They are also the most likely in the nation to go online on an average day, and they like to buy things online. Eighty-nine percent of online New Englanders used the Internet to find the answer to a specific question. Mid-Atlantic online users are shoppers and hobbyists. A high proportion of Mid-Atlantic users have college or graduate degrees (38%). Online residents of the Mid-Atlantic like to use the Internet to look for hobby information and are more likely to shop online than those in many other parts of the country (Spooner, 2003).

Online users in the National Capital Region are among the most experienced users in the country. They are wealthier and more educated than the national average. Many in this area are able to connect to the Internet from work and report using the Internet for work purposes. On the other hand, this region has the lowest rate of daily home Internet use. These users are more likely than their peers elsewhere in the nation to get news online, look for financial information, or seek help for their health (Spooner, 2003).

Southeastern Internet users are predominately home-based users who focus mostly on family and friends. On an average day, 80% of those who go online in the Southeast do so from home. These users feel more strongly than most others that the Internet has greatly enhanced their relationships with family and friends. They are among the least likely to shop online or look for information about hobbies online (Spooner, 2003). Similarly, online Southerners are primarily surfing in search of fun, news, and health information. This region has the lowest rate of Internet access of any region in the US and is the only region with fewer than half of adults online (48%). Southerners are less likely to use the Internet than their peers in just about every category. Yet, surfing the Web just for fun and getting news is quite popular among these users. In fact, online southerners are the most likely in the nation to have sought health information online (Spooner).

Internet users from the Industrial Midwest contain many novices who use the Internet to keep in touch with friends, while those from the Upper Midwest are predominately middle-aged, educated, and lukewarm about the Net. This region has one of the nation's smallest proportions of younger users (aged 18–24) (Spooner, 2003). In terms of those who are online and living in the Upper Midwest, they are much less likely than other Americans to credit the Internet with making improvements in their lives or about the Internet's impact on improving their connections with family and friends (Spooner). Those from the Lower Midwest are generally older, lower-income adults who use the Internet for fun and news (Spooner).

Online users from the Border States are often enthusiastic users in one of the most wired regions in the country. Their Southwest neighbors are among the most likely to get news or search for a job online and they are very enthusiastic about the positive effects of the Internet on their lives (Spooner, 2003).

Finally, regarding Internet users on the western seaboard, those from the Mountain States tend to be more experienced users who access the Internet from home more often that those in any other region. The region also has one of the smallest proportions of wealthy Internet users and the largest proportion of female users in the country (Spooner, 2003).

The Pacific Northwest has one of the largest cohorts of older users (aged 55+). This region's Internet users are experienced and are efficient when they are online – they are most likely to spend 30 min or less online on an average day. They are also less likely than their peers elsewhere to engage in many of the Web's more popular activities, with the exception of email (Spooner, 2003). Finally, Californian Internet users make up some of the most experienced regional user populations in the country. Users in California are among the wealthiest and most educated in the country. Californians lead the nation in the use of broadband (Spooner).

Gender-Based Utilization

The Internet was primarily used by men in its early days, but by 2000 and continuing on to today, the user population has divided more evenly. Younger women are more likely than younger men to be online, but older men are more likely than older women to be online (Fellows, 2005). Among seniors, 34% of men aged 65 and above use the Internet, compared with just 21% of women of that age (Fellows).

Interestingly, 60% of Black women are Internet users compared with only 50% of Black men. Unmarried men (62%) are more likely than unmarried women (56%) to be Internet users, while equal proportions of married women (75%) and married men (72%) go online (Fellows).

In general, on a typical day, men (61%) are slightly more likely to go online than women (57%) and they will do so more often during the day than women who are online (Fellows, 2005). Compared with women, online men are more likely to use the Internet to check the weather, get news, get do-it-yourself information, check for sports information, get political information, get financial information, do job-related research, download software, listen to or down load music, rate a product/person/service through an online reputation system, use a webcam, and take a class. On the other hand, online women are more likely to use the Internet to send and receive email, get maps and directions, look for health and medical information, use Web sites to get support for health or personal problems, and get religious information (Fellows). These findings suggest that men and women share an appreciation of what the Internet does for their lives, particularly in making their lives more efficient, and expanding their world of information. Men seem to value these strengths most in the context of the activities of their lives, from jobs to pastimes, while women seem to value them most in the context of the relationships with family, friends, colleagues, and communities. Finally, in terms of risks and security, men and women share concerns about personal risks and dangers from being online. But women express more fears than men about the Internet being a vehicle for national and worldwide problems such as criminal use of the Internet, child pornography, and terrorism (Fellows).

Children and the Internet

Children today are growing up in a remarkably different world than their parents. They are more connected than any preceding generation of human beings. While some of their parents and many of their grandparents are still learning about computers and the Internet, approximately 53 million children (91%) over the age of 3 use computers and another 35 million (35%) use the Internet (DeBell & Chapman, 2006). The use of these technologies starts early and only increases as they get older. Two-thirds of children in nursery school, 80% of kindergartners, and 97% of students in grades 9–12 use computers (DeBell & Chapman). In terms of Internet utilization, 23% of children in nursery school, 50% of third graders, and 79% of high school students use the Internet (DeBell & Chapman). While in the 1990s boys used computers and the Internet more than girls, by 2003, this lead had vanished (DeBell & Chapman).

There is significant variability in the way groups of kids use computers and the Internet. In 2003, 56% of students used home computers primarily to play games. On the other hand, approximately 47% use their computers to complete school assignments or connect to the Internet (DeBell & Chapman, 2006). About 62–69%

of students in grades 6–12 use home computers to complete school assignments, 54–64% to connect to the Internet, and 57–61% to play games.

As with adults, computer and Internet use among children is divided along demographic and socioeconomic lines. Unfortunately many disadvantaged students are only able to use the Internet at school. As may be expected, students with a physical disability are less likely than students without disabilities to use computers and the Internet (DeBell & Chapman, 2006). Children who live in families earning less that $20,000, students whose parents lack a high school diploma, and students who live in households where only Spanish is spoken are much less likely to use a computer or the Internet (DeBell & Chapman).

Teens and the Internet

The overwhelming majority (87% or 21 million) of US teens, aged 12–17, now use the Internet. This represents an increase from roughly 17 million in 2000. As their numbers have risen, so has the intensity with which teens use the Internet. Teenagers use the Internet more often and in a greater variety of ways than they did in 2000 (Lenhart, Madden, & Hitlin, 2005). There are now approximately 11 million teens who go online daily, compared to about 7 million in 2000. Wired teens are more frequent users of instant messaging and they are now more likely to play games online, make purchases, get news, and seek health information. On the other end of the spectrum, 13% of American teenagers (3 million teens) still do not use the Internet. Those teens who remain offline are most likely to be from low-income homes with limited access to technology. They are also more likely to be African-American (Lenhart et al.).

Most (84%) teens own at least one personal media device: a desktop or laptop computer, a cell phone, or a personal digital assistant (PDA). More than 40% of teens say they have two or more devices, while 12% have three, and 2% report having four electronic media devices. Only 16% of all teens report that they do not own any personal media device (Lenhart et al., 2005). In terms of what teens are doing with these devices, almost half of online teens (45%) own a cell phone, and 33% have used a cell phone to send a text message. Teens who own cell phones are most likely to use other online communication tools (Lenhart et al.). Text messaging (short messaging service or SMS) allows users to send messages of up to 160 characters from one personal technology or communications device to another. Text messaging is the preferred method of communication among teens, although many continue to use email, which they consider to be for "old people" (Lenhart et al.). Indeed, it appears that instant messaging has become the digital communication backbone of teens' daily lives. About half of instant-messaging teens (32% of *all* teens) use IM every single day. IM has become a routine part of teens' daily Internet diet and is used for many things like making plans with friends, discussing homework, joking around, and checking in with parents (Lenhart et al.). Almost half of all teenagers and in particular girls and those teens living in the urban environment own cell phones (Lenhart et al.). Despite these new technological realities, the landline telephone is a more favored communication medium. Even today spending more time physically with friends doing social things outside of school, occupies more of a teens time than does using technology. On an average, youth between ages 12–17 spend 10.3 h a week with friends doing social activities outside of school and about 7.8 h talking with friends via telephone, email, IM, or text messaging (Lenhart et al.).

Going to Junior High seems to be an important factor in using technology for many teens. Only 60% of the sixth graders report using the Internet, while 82% of seventh graders are online. In addition, older teenage girls (aged 15–17) use information and communication technologies the most. They are much more likely than boys and younger girls to use email, text messaging, search for information about prospective schools, seek health and religious information, and visit entertainment-related Web sites. Interestingly, overall 31% of all online teens (6 million teens) use the Internet to get health information (Lenhart et al., 2005).

Online Seniors

Approximately 8 million (22%) seniors over the age of 65 use the Internet (Fox, 2004). While online seniors are evenly divided between men and women, as a group, they are still made up predominately of Whites, highly educated seniors, and those living in households with higher incomes and who have Internet access (Fox). Email is equally popular among Internet users above and below the age of 65. Online seniors are using the Internet to accomplish a wide variety of activities. For example, 66% of online seniors looked for health or medical information or completed product research online. Almost half of online seniors purchased something online while 41% have made travel reservations online and 60% visited government Web sites. More than a quarter (26%) of wired seniors searched for religious and spiritual information and 20% conduct online banking transactions (Fox).

While wired seniors are transforming the notion of retiring, still most seniors (78%) are not using the Internet, do not know many people who use email or surf the Web, and cannot imagine why they would spend money and time learning how to use a computer (Fox, 2004). Because seniors are also more likely than any other age group to be living with some kind of disability, this may impact their desire or ability to obtain computer training or otherwise become computer savvy (Fox).

Generational Influences

As outlined above, young Internet users have embraced the Internet and use it primarily for communication, creativity, and social uses. Teens and Generation Y (age 18–28) are the most likely to send and receive instant messages, play online games, create blogs, download music, and search for school information. Interestingly, this does not appear to be an issue related to broadband access. Internet users in their thirties are about as likely as users in their 20s to have broadband at home but they are much less likely than younger users to use the Internet for games and IM (Fox & Madden, 2005). Also, adult Internet users are more likely than Internet users in other age groups to engage in online financial transactions. While Internet users with home broadband access are most likely to do these activities, fully 50% of all Internet users between 29 and 40 years old bank online, compared to 38% of Internet users between the ages of 18–28 (Fox & Madden).

Despite these well-recognized differences in Internet use associated with age, almost all (90%) Internet users send or receive email. This is somewhat surprising given the discussion above relating to age-related differences among those online. Email is even the most popular online activity for seniors. However, the best place to reach someone aged 70 and older is still offline. On the other hand, buying a product online is also equally popular with all Internet users except among teens and seniors over the age 70 (Fox & Madden, 2005). Thus, as can be seen, while there is some intergenerational variability, many activities of online users tend to fit into relatively discreet age-related or generational patterns. Despite this reality, a few activities (email) span generations and others (online shopping) do not cross well-recognized age or generational lines.

Internet Enablers

Several factors have likely contributed to the tremendous growth of the Internet over the last decade. Two factors, home broadband adoption and wireless access may be particularly important. The number of Americans who have broadband at home increased 40% from 60 million in March 2005 to 84 million in March 2006. This single year increase doubles the 20% increase in the rate of broadband adoption that was seen from 2004 to 2005 (Horrigan, 2006). Much of the increase is due to new Internet users who have bypassed dial-up connections and gone straight to high-speed connections. Interestingly, the growth in broadband adoption has been particularly strong in middle-income households, especially among African-Americans and those with little education. For example, broadband adoption grew by 68% since March 2005 among people living in households with incomes between $40,000 and $50,000 per year while adoption among African-Americans increased by 121% in the same time period (Horrigan, 2006). In addition, home high-speed adoption also grew rapidly among those with less than a high-school education (by 70%) and senior citizens (by 63%) while the pace of adoption in rural areas was also brisk (39%) (Horrigan, 2006).

High speed Internet connections appear to draw people deeper into Internet use. More than half of online users (53%) say they spend more time online since getting a high-speed Internet connection at home (Horrigan, 2006). In addition, 35% (48 million adults) of Internet users report posting online content to the Web with home broadband users accounting for 73% of those who post content to the Internet. As such, there appears to be a significant association between having a home broadband connection and users putting content online (Horrigan, 2006). With so many Americans having home high-speed Internet access, user-generated content is no longer only possible for high-income broadband users (Horrigan, 2006).

Wireless Internet access is another phenomenon facilitating rapid Internet adoption. Approximately 34% of Internet users have logged onto the Internet via a wireless device (Horrigan, 2007). Like broadband utilization, wireless access users, especially when checking email and getting news, tend to be more deeply engaged in cyber activities than those without wireless access (Horrigan, 2007). Almost three quarters (72%) of wireless Internet users check email on a typical day compared with 63% of home broadband and 54% of all Internet users (Horrigan, 2007). Similarly, 46% of wireless users get news online compared with 38 and 31% of home broadband and all Internet users, respectively (Horrigan, 2007).

In terms of where and how people are wirelessly accessing the Internet, more than one quarter (27%) of Internet users overall access the net wirelessly at a place other than home or work. In addition, almost 40% of Internet users have a laptop computer and almost 90% of laptop users connect to the Internet via a home wireless network (Horrigan, 2007). Another 25% of Internet users own Web-enabled cell phones. Approximately half (54%) of these cell phone users use their phones to access the Internet. With respect to PDAs, some 13% of Internet users own PDAs that can connect to the Internet. About 82% of these Internet users have used their PDAs to connect to the Web (Horrigan, 2007).

Finally, the tremendous growth in the number of individuals using the Internet, the growth in the ways in which they access the Internet, and the growth in the depth and intensity with which they are using the Internet have spawned the development of several related technologies and applications. These include things like spam or unsolicited bulk commercial email, spyware or programs that are loaded onto computer devices without the owner's consent and track the user's online activities. Internet phishing which is unsolicited email that attempt to acquire sedative user information by pretending to be a trustworthy person or business and RSS which is a file format that enables the syndication of Web content to specific subscribers, are also outgrowths of widespread Internet use (Rainie, 2005). Large numbers of Internet users do not know what some of these things are. While most (>50%) of Internet users have a good idea of Spam, Firewalls, Spyware, Internet cookies, and adware, most (>50%) are not really sure or have never heard of phishing, podcasting, or RSS feeds (Rainie). With all the realized and potential benefits the Internet has to offer, this data suggest that technology, in some cases, may be ahead of the public's awareness of both the technology and the potential hazards or dangers (Rainie). Not surprisingly, as with several of the other categories of Internet users, men, individuals with college degrees, younger Internet users, and those who use the Internet often are the most likely to be familiar with these issues and concepts.

Summary

In less than 15 years since the widespread availability of the first Web browser from Netscape, Internet utilization has rapidly increased and evolved. While in the early days most Internet users were wealthy males, many more in the middle and lower classes are now online and the gender gap has disappeared. Several relatively discreet regional Internet user profiles can even be constructed. In terms of age, children are much more connected than their parents and grandparents. They also tend to use the Internet in a much broader array of ways than older users. Interestingly though, email remains the single most popular online activity among all age groups. The poor, less educated and minorities, particularly African-Americans, tend to be the least well connected to the Internet.

References

DeBell, M., & Chapman, C. (2006). *Computer and Internet use by students in 2003*. Washington, DC: US Department of Education, National Center for Education Statistics.

Fellows, D. (2005). *How women and men use the Internet*. Washington, DC: Pew Charitable Trusts.

Fox, S. (2004). *Older Americans and the Internet*. Washington, DC: Pew Charitable Trusts.

Fox, S., & Madden, M. (2005). *Generations online*. Washington, DC: Pew Charitable Trusts.

Horrigan, J. (2006). *Home broadband adoption*. Washington, DC: Pew Charitable Trusts.

Horrigan, J. (2007). *Wireless Internet access*. Washington, DC: Pew Charitable Trusts.

Lenhart, A., Madden, M., & Hitlin, P. (2005). *Teens and technology*. Washington, DC: Pew Charitable Trusts.

Madden, M. (2007). *Internet penetration and impact, April 2006*. Washington, DC: Pew Charitable Trusts.

Rainie, L. (2005). *Data memo: Internet terminology*. www.pewInternet.org [On-line].

Rainie, L., Fox, S., Horrigan, J., Fellows, D., Lenhart, A., Madden, M., et al. (2005). *Internet: The mainstreaming of online life*. Washington, DC: Pew Charitable Trusts.

Spooner, T. (2003). *Internet use by region in the US*. Washington, DC: Pew Charitable Trusts.

7
The iHealth Revolution

Michael Christopher Gibbons

Even as the increasing prominence and pervasiveness of the Internet is causing significant changes in many aspects of society, it is also causing significant shifts in the way people think, talk, and act regarding their health and health care. The changes are suggesting such fundamental shifts in the way people experience and providers practice health and health care that it may be best characterized as an iHealth (Internet-Health) revolution. This chapter will discuss the impact of the Internet on the health and healthcare experiences of patients.

Early Online Health Patterns and Practices

As early as the year 2000, just 6 years after the widespread availability of the first Web browser, 52 million Americans had used the Web to get health or medical information (Fox et al., 2000). Overall, these health seekers found their online experiences to be satisfying. Forty-eight percent of these health seekers thought that the advice they found helped them improve the way they take care of themselves and 55% say Internet access has improved the way they get medical information (Fox et al.). Almost all health seekers (92%) found the information useful and 81% learned something new (Fox et al.). Almost half (43%) of health seekers were using the Internet to search for health or medical information for themselves and another 54% were searching on behalf of someone else. Fifty percent of those that were seeing online health information for themselves indicated that the information influenced the way they eat and exercise (Fox et al.). In terms of more specific impact of online health information, 70% of the 21 million people who in the year 2000 reported that Web-based health information had impacted them, reported that it affected their decision about how to treat an illness or condition, 50% said it led them to ask a doctor new questions or get a second opinion while 28% said the information affected their decision about whether or not to visit a doctor at all (Fox et al.).

In these "early" days of online health seeking, most people (91%) were looking for information regarding a physical illness or mental health (26%) issue. Only 13% of online health seekers at that time had sought information about fitness or nutrition, 11% about healthcare news, and only 9% had sought information about specific doctors (Fox et al., 2000). It appears that at this time, in terms of health, the Internet was more a disease or illness research tool than anything else. On the one hand, only 9% of health seekers had communicated with providers online and only 10% had purchased medicines or gotten medical advice from an online doctor. Slightly more people (21%) had given their email address to a health-oriented Web site or (17%) provided their name or other personal information to a health Web site (Fox et al.). In addition to being a health research tool, the Internet enabled family members to have a convenient method for getting "second opinions" regarding health issues for ailing family and friends (Fox et al.).

Shifting Online Health Norms

Over the next 3 years, online health information seeking behaviors began to change in several significant ways. Probably the most notable change was a 2-year 62% increase (73 million) in the number of people who were using the Internet for health purposes (Fox & Rainie, 2002). On any given day, 6 million Americans would be online seeking medical advice. By this time, Americans were seeking for much more than information about diseases or illnesses. They were looking for information about prescription drugs, exploring weight loss programs, and preparing for upcoming doctor's appointments (Fox & Rainie). In 2002, the typical health seeker started a search at a search engine, not a health Web site. Health seekers also visited 2–5 health sites during an average 30-min session. Often they found what they were looking for, felt reassured by the information, and were subsequently bringing this information to upcoming physician office visits to discuss it with their doctors (Fox & Rainie). At the same time there seemed to be less concern among health seekers regarding the quality of health information they were finding online. In 2000, 86% of health seekers were concerned about getting unreliable health information and 58% of health seekers actually checked into the authors of online health information. By 2002, however, only about 25% thoroughly checked online health sources and very few (2%) reported suffering from harmful effects out of acting on bad health information they found on the Web (Fox & Rainie).

By 2002, these online health seekers appear to have become more Internet health savvy in that 73% of health seekers had at some point rejected health information provided online. Almost half (47%) of health seekers decided not to use the health information because the Web site seemed too commercial and implied greater concern for profits than accuracy of information. Forty-two percent decided not to use some online health information because they could not verify the source of the information and 37% did not use the information because they could not determine when the information had been last updated (Fox & Rainie, 2002). Some online health seekers also used certain visual Web cues to decide if they should use online health information. These online health seekers would generally not use information if there was no obvious "seal of approval" on the Web site, if the Web site was sloppily or unprofessionally designed, or if in the opinion of the health seeker (or their own doctor) the Web site contained bad information (Fox & Rainie). Despite the emergence of a growing number of unconcerned online health seekers, most were still relying on their doctor as a primary guidance and for fact checking of health information found online. They seemed to be supplementing their care with information obtained from the Web and using this information to help clarify information that remained unclear after a doctor's appointment (Fox & Rainie).

In general, most physicians seemed to be responding positively to these new "informed" patients. Almost 80% of patients who talked to their doctor about health information obtained online reports that their doctors were very much or somewhat interested in (Fox & Rainie, 2002). These online health seekers seemed to be finding the right information. Fully 82% of online health seekers who shared online information with their providers said the doctor or nurse agreed with the information. Only 13% of online health seekers who shared the information with their doctors received negative feedback from their doctors regarding the information (Fox & Rainie).

Although there had been little change between 2000 and 2002 in the proportion (9%) of online health seekers who had participated in online health communication with providers, 90% of online health seekers said they would like to be able to email their doctors, if their doctors responded in a timely fashion and 37% said they would be willing to pay for it (Fox & Rainie, 2002).

Online support groups began to emerge as another Internet-based health resource. Only 10% of online health seekers chose to participate in these support groups or disease-oriented email list serves in 2002 (Fox & Rainie, 2002). It appears that privacy concerns and the need for a "human connection" kept more online health seekers from using these types of services (Fox & Rainie). While most online health seekers tend not to use these services, those who do are most in need and may be more likely to use these services than their healthier counterparts. Ten percent of health seekers in fair or poor health used an online support group the last time they went online, compared with only 1% of those in excellent health. In addition, 14% of online health seekers in fair or poor health have ever used these types of services while only 5% of those in excellent health have done so (Fox & Rainie). Finally, only 8% of health seekers have set up personal profiles at a favorite health Web site or customized a health portal so that only they received specific health information. Many more, however, have signed up for an electronic email health newsletter (Fox & Rainie).

The growth and development of the "informed health seeker" continued through 2003 when 80% of adult Internet users or about 93 million people reported searching online for health information (Fox & Fallows, 2003). Not only had the raw number of people engaging in online health activities continued to substantially increase, but also the variety of online health topics being considered burgeoned to the extent that the act of seeking online health information became the third most popular online activity behind email and consumer product research (Fox & Fallows). The growing variety of topics searched online included, among others, specific disease or medical problems (63%), medical treatments and procedures (47%), diet, nutrition-related information (44%), exercise or fitness (36%), prescription or over-the-counter medicines (34%), and alternative treatments and medicines (28%) (Fox & Fallows). Many health seekers report that this ability seems to supplement their knowledge empowerment. It also enabled them to ask better questions of their doctors and to have less fear of the unknown (Fox & Fallows).

In addition to the change in attitudes, behaviors, and perceptions of patients, there appeared to be some evidence of an evolution of physician attitudes toward the "increasingly informed patients." Generally speaking, those patients who discussed online health information with their providers found them to be either "partners in the care process" or more paternalistic and disinterested (Fox & Fallows, 2003). While not all physicians can be accurately characterized by one of these two positions, some could. Indeed, even as the American Medical Association was warning patients about the risk of online health information, many doctors reported using the Internet themselves to supplement their medical knowledge and the care they provide to patients (Fox & Rainie, 2002).

Despite a slow start, online health seekers were increasingly turning to health-oriented email lists and online support groups for emotional support. By 2003, 32 million Americans or 30% of email users had sent or received health-related email. Approximately 50% of email users exchanged health-related emails with family members or friends and 7% had done so with a doctor or provider (Fox & Rainie, 2002). Fully 90% of people engaging in health-related email exchange found this activity useful (Fox & Rainie). Most online health seekers found health-related email exchanges useful because it helped in connecting them to needed emotional support as well as to needed practical help and insight from others in similar situations (Fox & Fallows, 2003; Fox & Rainie). Some online health seekers found support by giving (rather than seeking) first hand knowledge about a particular illness or by helping others keep up with new advances and breaking news regarding health topics of mutual interest (Fox & Rainie). This may be of particular importance because some online health seekers appear to be unaware of currently available Web health resources including drug interaction information, diagnostic tools and symptom finders, test results, information for caregivers, and connections to local health resources (Fox & Fallows).

Contemporary Online Health Trends

In response to the increasing online health-consumer demand, online search engines responded. While a plethora of Web sites containing health information about diseases, health conditions, medical treatments, or surgical procedures continued to grow, by 2005, the largest growth was seen in the areas of diet, fitness, exercise, and over-the-counter medicines (Fox, 2005). In addition, substantial growth was also seen in the number of searches regarding health insurance, specific doctors, hospital services, and track records (Fox, 2005). As such, approximately 113 million people or 80% of adult Internet users report having used the Internet to search for health information (Fox, 2006). In addition, the number of Internet users with a high school diploma who have looked for health information online has surged to 71%.

To date, 66% of all health searches begin at a search engine like Google or Yahoo with younger online health seekers being most likely to use these starting points (Fox, 2006). Women are more likely to be online health seekers and they are more likely to be searching for information on behalf of someone else (Fox, 2006). Almost 60% of online health seekers today visit at least two sites in a typical session and 33% of these individuals later talk to a doctor about what they found online (Fox, 2006).

In terms of the provider community, there now appears to be some concern over whether these large numbers of online health seekers are self-diagnosing and self-medicating based on information they find online, without consulting medical providers (Fox, 2006). In actuality, patients who searched online for themselves were more likely to discuss online information with a provider than those who were searching online for someone else (Fox, 2006). The importance of this is highlighted by the fact that currently 50% of all health searches are done on behalf of someone else (Fox, 2006). While most people find online health information useful, most indicate that it only has a minor impact on actual healthcare choices for themselves or the way they care for someone else (Fox, 2006). The exception to this rule is among those who have recently received a serious diagnosis or experienced some other health crisis within the last year. Fourteen percent of these individuals indicate that their last search had a major impact on a health decision compared to only 7% of those without a major health experience in the last year (Fox, 2006).

Finally, today approximately 75% of all online health seekers do not routinely check the quality of the health information they find on the Web. In part this may be due to the substantial increase in the numbers of lower educated consumers who are now searching for health information online. Health seekers with less education are not as likely to check the quality of online health information as compared to more highly educated online health seekers (Fox, 2006).

Summary

Since the early days of the Internet, the numbers of online health seekers have swelled to approximately 113 million people. During this time, significant shifts in the practices and habits of online health seekers were evident. These individuals increasingly became informed and empowered. This, at times, led to some friction with some healthcare providers. Over time, however, many providers themselves began using the Internet to enhance their medical knowledge and patient care services. The rapid growth in online health activities was fueled in part by significant increases in home broadband and wireless access which in turn enabled many health seekers to engage in much more intense health information seeking activities. Patients are drawn to the convenience and anonymity of online health information. They have generally been able to find what they are looking for and report that the Internet is increasingly helping them to connect to emotional support and practical help for dealing with their health issues. The Internet also provides many online opportunities to provide support by helping other online health seekers keep up with the latest information and health news. As the Internet has matured, there has been an increasing interest in wellness activities, information, and resources in addition to disease-oriented information and resources. Finally, the typical online health seeker is female. She is likely to search for information on behalf of a family member or friend, has a relatively easy time finding what she needs, and is often reassured and more confident as a result of getting the information and is in general, pleased with her online searching experience.

References

Fox, S. (2005). *Health information online*. Washington, DC: Pew Charitable Trusts.

Fox, S. (2006). *Online health search 2006*. Washington, DC: Pew Charitable Trusts.

Fox, S., & Fallows, D. (2003). *Internet health resources*. Washington, DC: Pew Charitable Trusts.

Fox, S., & Rainie, L. (2002). *Vital decisions: How internet users decide what information to trust when they or their loved ones are sick*. Washington, DC: Pew Charitable Trusts.

Fox, S., Rainie, L., Horrigan, J., Lenhart, A., Spooner, T., Burke, M., et al. (2000). *The online health care revolution: How the web helps Americans take better care of themselves*. Washington, DC: Pew Charitable Trusts.

8
Digital Disparities

Michael Christopher Gibbons

Since the mid-1990s when the World Wide Web became a powerful part of America's communications and information culture, there has been great concern that the nation's racial minorities and other underserved and disadvantaged populations would be further disadvantaged because Internet access was not spreading as quickly in the African-American community as it was in the White community. Former Assistant Secretary of Commerce, Larry Irving, said the following in his introduction to "Falling Through the Net," the 1999 Department of Commerce Study on the digital divide (the divide between those with access to new information technologies and those without): ["The digital divide" is now one of America's leading economic and civil rights issues] (US Department of Commerce, 1999a).

The basis for the secretary's assertion can be found in US telecommunications policy. The National Telecommunications and Information Administration (NTIA) is within the US Department of Commerce and functions as the US president's principal advisory body on telecommunications policy (US Department of Commerce, 1995). A fundamental premise of US telecommunications policy is the notion that all Americans should have access to affordable telephone service (universal service). Prior to this point, the most commonly used measure of universal service was "telephone penetration" or the percentage of all households in America that have a telephone on the premises (US Department of Commerce, 1995). However, significant growth in personal computer ownership and Internet access (see Chaps. 6 and 7) suggested the need to go beyond telephone penetration as a metric of universal access (US Department of Commerce, 1995). To accomplish this goal, the NTIA contracted with the Census Bureau to include questions regarding computer/modem ownership and usage in the Bureau's Current Population Survey, and to cross tab this information via several geodemographic characteristics (US Department of Commerce, 1995). This chapter will discuss the evidence and evolution of the digital divide in the US.

African-Americans and the Digital Divide

Based on this new data, the first report entitled "Falling through the net: A survey of the 'Have Nots' in rural and urban America," found that, in general the information "have nots" could disproportionately be found in the country's rural *and* urban inner cities (US Department of Commerce, 1995). While it was not surprising that lower income individuals as a group have difficulties connecting to the nation's information infrastructure, prior to this time it was not known that the areas of lowest telephone penetration existed in our nation's inner cities (US Department of Commerce). However, individuals living in rural communities had the lowest overall rates of computer ownership and Internet access (US Department of Commerce). In terms of race, Native Americans, Hispanics, and Blacks had the lowest rates of telephone penetration and computer/modem ownership. Finally, at that time, the single most seriously disadvantaged group were householders under the age of 25, in terms of both telephone penetration and computer/modem ownership (US Department of Commerce). Thus although, overall, the number of Americans connected to the nation's information infrastructure via telephone or Internet was soaring, a significant divide existed between Whites and minorities, rural and urban inner city dwellers, the poor and the young, in terms of telephone penetration and access to the Internet (US Department of Commerce).

A follow-up study done by the NTIA in 1997 revealed that although as a nation, Americans were rapidly embracing the Information Age through home electronic access, the disparities between the connected and unconnected in both telephone penetration, computer/modem ownership, and Internet access, persisted and appeared to be *widening* over time (US Department of Commerce, 1998). Additionally, for the first time, profiles of the least-connected groups began to emerge. They include the rural poor who have the lowest telephone penetration rates, rural and inner city minorities, particularly African-Americans and Hispanics, who have the lowest computer ownership rates, and female single parent households (US Department of Commerce, 1998). By 1999, those living in urban households with incomes over $75,000 were 20 times more likely to have Internet access than those living in rural poverty (US Department of Commerce, 1999a). Whites also became more likely to access the Internet from home than African-Americans no matter where they lived and the magnitude of these disparities seemed to be increasing (US Department of Commerce, 1999a).

Interestingly, several changes began to occur in the year 2000 that continue even today. The gap in basic Internet access between rural and urban households began to shrink. Also, Internet access among middle income and low educational level households began to surge (US Department of Commerce, 2000). In terms of computer ownership, the disparities between African-Americans and Whites were still large but had stabilized and not increased (US Department of Commerce, 2000).

As researchers began to try to explain the reasons for these differences, they found that among African-Americans, educational and income differences could not fully explain the identified disparities (US Department of Commerce, 2000). Further research began to highlight other important differences. In general, when compared to online Whites, online African-Americans are more likely to be women. They are also more likely to be from lower income households and least likely to have college degrees (Spooner & Rainie, 2005). Online African-Americans appear to be fairly young. Fifty-six percent of online Blacks are under the age of 34 and another 38% are between 35 and 54. In comparison, 40% of online Whites are under 35 and 46% are between the ages of 35 and 54 (Spooner & Rainie). One other prominent demographic feature of the African-American online population is that there are a lot of parents with children under 18. About 53% of online Blacks have a child under the age of 18 at home, while 42% of online Whites are parents of children of that age (Spooner & Rainie).

While there are similarities, it appears that African-Americans and Whites have differing online habits when surfing the net. Online Blacks are more likely to use the Internet for employment, job training, school research, to hunt for a place to live, and for entertainment purposes (Spooner & Rainie, 2005). African-Americans are significantly more likely to be engaged with online multimedia tools, looked at or listened to an online video or audio clip, played an online game and they are more likely to have downloaded music from the Web (Spooner & Rainie).

In contrast, the online behavior of Whites and African-Americans is similar when searching for general information. Both have used the Web in similar proportions to get general news, political news, to research product information, and to get travel information (Spooner & Rainie, 2005). Online Whites appear more likely to have sought financial information and to have checked out weather reports when online (Spooner & Rainie). They (online Whites) are also more than twice as likely as online Blacks to have participated in Web-based auctions and are much more likely to have bought products on the Internet (Spooner & Rainie). One significant difference is in the area of online religious and spiritual information. Online Blacks are 65% more likely to have sought such material on the Web than online Whites. This is particularly true among African-American women over age 30. Finally, both races are equally as likely to have done banking online, made a travel reservation, and bought or sold stocks (Spooner & Rainie).

Compared to African-American men, African-American women are much more likely to have obtained online health information, looked on the Web for job information, and sought spiritual or religious material online. African-American men, on the other hand, are more likely than women to have used the Web to seek financial data, purchase goods, and get sports information (Spooner & Rainie, 2005).

Overall, the reality is that the Internet has not yet become as essential or appealing a tool to online African-Americans as it has to online Whites. Just 36% of Blacks with Internet access go online on a typical day while 56% of Whites with Internet access are online on an average day. Whites and Blacks even have differing attitudes toward the Internet with online African-Americans not being as fervent in their appreciation of the Internet as online Whites (Spooner & Rainie, 2005). For example, while 73% of online Whites say they would miss the Internet if they could no longer access it, only 62% of online African-Americans say they would miss it. On the other hand, only 10% of online Whites say they would not miss the Internet at all if they were to lose access while 20% of online Blacks say the same thing.

Fifty percent of all White Internet users would miss email a lot if they could no longer use it, but only 39% of Black users agreed (Spooner & Rainie).

In terms of where they access the Internet, African-Americans Internet users are somewhat more likely than Whites to have their Internet access come exclusively through their jobs. Some 18% of African-American Internet users *only* have access to the Web at work, while 12% of White users are in that position.

Finally, while online privacy has become a significant concern for a majority of Internet users, African-Americans tend to be less trusting than Whites. They are also more concerned about their online privacy than Whites (Spooner & Rainie, 2005). These heightened privacy concerns are reflected in what they choose to do online. Online African-Americans are less likely to participate in high-trust activities like auctions or to give their credit card information to an online vendor. They are also less likely than White Internet users to trade their personal information for access to a Web site. Yet African-Americans still engage in online banking, making travel arrangements, or trading stocks online. In addition Black Internet users have been found to be more likely than White Internet users to have made a friend online (Spooner & Rainie).

Online Latinos

With the rapid rise in the US Latino population over the last decade, there have come new opportunities for demographers, survey researchers, and others to enhance our knowledge about many facets of Latinos living in America. In the fall of 2006, the Pew Hispanic Center conducted a survey of over 6,000 Latino adults with landline telephones (Fox & Livingston, 2007). According to the results of this survey 56% of Latinos in the US use the Internet. This compares to 71% of non-Hispanic Whites and 60% of non-Hispanic Blacks who use the Internet (Fox & Livingston). Seventy-eight percent of English-speaking Latinos and 76% of bilingual Latinos use the Internet. Only 32% of Spanish-only-speaking Latinos use the Internet. In addition, more than three quarters (76%) of US-born Latinos go online, compared with 43% of those born outside the US. Similarly 80% of second-generation Latinos and 71% of third-generation Latinos go online. Almost 90% of Latinos with a college degree go online, whereas only 31% of those without a high school diploma go online. Also Mexicans are the largest national origin group in the US Latino population and are among the least likely groups to go online; only 52% of Mexican Latinos use the Internet (Fox & Livingston).

As in the general population, certain groups of Latinos are less likely than others to go online. In particular, those with less education, those with lower household incomes, and those who are over the age of 60 are least likely to be online (Fox & Livingston, 2007). As discussed in the previous chapters, home broadband connections increase the intensity with which online seekers use the Internet. Overall, 29% of Hispanic adults have home broadband connections, compared with 43% of White adults. This is, in part, due to the fact that Latino Internet users are less likely than non-Hispanic White Internet users to have any kind of Internet connection at home (79% compared to 92%) (Fox & Livingston).

Interestingly, among Latinos, the information and communications revolution is not limited to the computer screen. Some Latinos who do not use the Internet are connecting to the communications superhighway via cell phone (Fox & Livingston, 2007). Almost sixty percent (59%) of Latino adults have a cell phone and 49% of Latino cell phone users send and receive text messages on their phone. Only 18% of Latino adults have a cell phone but do not go online. Roughly one quarter (26%) of Latino adults have neither a cell phone nor an Internet connection (Fox & Livingston).

Online Asian-Americans

In stark contrast to other racial and ethnic groups Asian-Americans who speak English are the most wired racial or ethnic group in America. They are also the Internet's heaviest and most experienced users (Spooner & Rainie, 2001). Over 5 million Asian-Americans (75%) have used the Internet. This compares to 58% of Whites, 43% of African-Americans, and 50% of English-speaking Hispanics (Spooner & Rainie). With 70% of Asian-Americans on line, on any given day they are the most avid daily users of the Internet in the nation (Spooner & Rainie).

Typically, Asians spend more time online than other racial and ethnic groups. In addition, they engage the Internet at a much higher level of intensity on a typical day than other groups and as such the Internet represents an extremely important and fundamental component of daily living for Asian-Americans (Spooner & Rainie, 2001). In terms of specific online activities, online Asian-Americans are much more likely than others to get information about financial matters, travel, and political information or to use the Internet as an educational or employment resource (Spooner & Rainie).

There are some interesting gender differences among online Asian-Americans. Overall Asian-American men engage in online activities more than Asian-American women. Asian-American women enjoy the entertainment-oriented activities available on the Internet. These include finding information about hobbies, listening to music, getting sports information, and shopping (Spooner & Rainie, 2001). On the other hand, Asian-American men prefer financial information, travel information, and political news (Spooner & Rainie).

The Future of Digital Disparities

If nothing else, the previous discussion highlights the fact that digital disparities are complex, nuanced, and multifaceted. The underlying causes of these disparities cannot be fully explained by socioeconomic and geographic factors. Much more research is needed for us to go beyond binary characterizations of Internet user demographics and attitudes to more completely understand the determinants of utilization, the implications of differential utilization patterns, and, most importantly, how we can build upon this knowledge to take advantage of the Internet revolution to ensure equitable utilization and maximize beneficial health outcomes. If recent history is any barometer of future activity, the nature and magnitude of these digital disparities is likely to change. Some may diminish in magnitude or relevance while others may increase. Indeed other disparities that are not currently recognized or existent may arise.

As information technology plays an ever-increasing role in Americans' economic and social lives, the potential health implications of these findings need to be more clearly evaluated because the prospect that some people will be left behind in the information age may have serious repercussions (US Department of Commerce, 1999b). Persistent digital disparities in access or utilization could leave some groups less able to take advantage of cutting edge innovations in population health technologies that enhance disease surveillance, environmental monitoring, food safety, emergency planning, disaster management, and geographic information systems-based tracking of environmental hazards (Eng, 2004). In the end, by moving away from the desire for dichotomous explications of Internet use among specific population groups, and building on a notion of the digital disparity spectrum (Lenhart & Horrigan, 2003) in access, utilization, in determinants and health outcomes, it may significantly enhance our understanding of this phenomenon and enable quantum leaps forward in the design and diffusion of novel electronic innovations developed to help address inequalities in Internet access, utilization, and ultimately, healthcare outcomes.

References

Eng, T. R. (2004). Population health technologies: Emerging innovations for the health of the public. *American Journal of Preventive Medicine, 26*, 237–242.

Fox, S., & Livingston, G. (2007). *Latinos online*. Washington, DC: Pew Charitable Trusts.

Lenhart, A., & Horrigan, J. (2003). Revisualizing the digital divide as a digital spectrum. *IT and Society, 1*, 23–39.

Spooner, T., & Rainie, L. (2001). *Asian Americans and the Internet*. Washington, DC: Pew Charitable Trusts.

Spooner, T., & Rainie, L. (2005). *African-Americans and the internet*. Washington, DC: Pew Internet & American Life Project.

US Department of Commerce, N. T. a. I. A. (1995). *Falling through the net: A survey of the "Have nots" in urban and rural America*. Washington, DC: GPO.

US Department of Commerce, N. T. a. I. A. (1998). *Falling through the net II: New data on the digital divide*. Washington, DC: GPO.

US Department of Commerce, N. T. a. I. A. (1999a). *Falling through the net: Defining the digital divide*. Washington, DC: GPO.

US Department of Commerce, N. T. a. I. A. (1999b). The digital divide summit. http://www.ntia. doc.gov/ntiahome/digitaldivide/summit/[On-line].

US Department of Commerce, N. T. a. I. A. (2000). *Falling through the net: Towards digital inclusion*. Washington, DC: GPO.

Section III

9
The Role of eHealth in Patient Engagement and Quality Improvement

David Ahern, Judith M. Phalen, and Charles B. Eaton

Introduction

Despite accounting for 16% of annual Gross Domestic Product (Anderson, Frogner, Johns, & Reinhardt, 2006), the $1.88 trillion American healthcare system does not rank among the top nations of the world on several key dimensions with respect to healthcare quality, including infant mortality and healthy life expectancy (Schoen, Davis, How, & Schoenbaum, 2006; The Commonwealth Fund Commission on a High Performance Health System, 2006). Although a recent report from the National Committee on Quality Assurance (NCQA) describes improvements in preventive services and treatments known to enhance chronic disease management for people enrolled in health plans (National Committee for Quality Assurance, 2006), consistent evidence indicates that for most health conditions for which there are established evidence-based standards of care, Americans receive those treatments only about 50% of the time (Asch et al., 2006; McGlynn et al., 2003). Recently, Wennberg, Fisher, Sharp, McAndrew, and Bronner (2006) demonstrated the substantial regional variation in practice patterns and outcomes with respect to quality of care for Medicare recipients. Notably, the quality of care observed in regions with excess capacity of hospital and provider resources, and which were perceived as exemplary, was no better than regions with lesser capacity or reputation, and in some cases for certain conditions, worse. Hence, consumers increasingly are becoming worried about the relentless growth in healthcare costs year-to-year and about quality and safety issues (ABC News/USA TODAY/Kaiser Family Foundation health care poll, 2006). However, their primary concern is reducing the cost of their health insurance premiums (ABC News/USA TODAY/ Kaiser Family Foundation health care poll; Harris Interactive, 2005a).

Access to quality care also appears to be uneven across socioeconomic and racial subgroups (Liu et al., 2006). African-American and Hispanic populations continue to fare worse than their Caucasian counterparts in terms of access to services and evidence-based care, although improvements have been observed recently (Agency for Healthcare Research and Quality, 2005). Moreover, the variation in quality of care may be less among different sociodemographic and racial groups than the gap which exists between observed and desirable quality for all groups (Asch et al.,

2006). Nevertheless, health disparities remain a major dilemma for the healthcare system (Trivedi, Zaslavsky, Schneider, & Ayanian, 2006).

The current and ongoing challenges of quality and access serve as the backdrop for a discussion of the potential for eHealth to both improve healthcare quality for all Americans, and increase meaningful access for traditionally underserved populations. The ability of eHealth applications to engage and activate diverse patients through (1) content and approaches that take into account personal demographics such as age, ethnicity, gender, and race; (2) salient and timely messaging and reminders for such things as self-care behaviors (e.g., taking medications, monitoring blood glucose levels), appointments scheduling/follow-up, and health screenings (e.g., mammograms, blood pressure); (3) support for self-management (e.g., programs for disease management, weight loss, and smoking cessation); and (4) social support, are the major premises of this chapter. What follows is a focused review of eHealth with particular attention paid to how these applications can meaningfully engage and activate patients to become more informed about their health and skilled in self-management, thereby stimulating better performance and improved quality from the healthcare system.

We will use the terms "consumer" and "patient" somewhat interchangeably throughout the chapter to accommodate the various roles that individuals may assume with respect to their health status and use of the healthcare system.

Definition and Perceptions of eHealth

For the purposes of this chapter, eHealth is defined as the use of emerging interactive technologies (i.e., Internet, interactive TV, interactive voice response systems, kiosks, Internet-enabled cell phones and personal digital assistants [PDAs], CD-ROMs, DVDs) to enable health improvement and healthcare services (Eng, 2001). This widely accepted definition accommodates eHealth applications for patients and providers, as well as more infrastructure-related programs, e.g., electronic medical records (EMRs) and personal health records (PHRs).

Eighty-seven percent of American Internet users believe that they find reliable healthcare information online (Harris Interactive, 2006a), with 80% of them having searched for information on health topics including medical treatments, environmental health hazards, mental health, and problems with substance use (Fox, 2006). The majority of Web users in France, Germany, and Japan believe that online healthcare information is trustworthy and of good quality, and a sizeable portion of those populations think that the Internet will improve relationships with their doctors (Taylor, 2002). Most online adults in the US believe that the use of EMRs will reduce the frequency of medical errors, lower healthcare costs, and improve the quality of care by eliminating redundant or unnecessary procedures (Harris Interactive, 2005b). In addition, the majority of US adults, both online and offline, favor the adoption of new medical technologies by their doctors (e.g., EMRs, home monitoring devices, electronic messaging) (Harris Interactive, 2005c). Hence, most consumers hold a positive opinion about the importance of the Internet and other technologies for health-related purposes, as well as a desire to have increased access to these eHealth applications (Harris Interactive, 2006b). Clearly, patients view the Internet as a primary source of health information, supplementing the information and recommendations they receive from their physicians (Horrigan & Rainie, 2002). Nevertheless, patients continue to consider their physicians as the most reliable and credible source of health information and medical advice, thereby highlighting the importance of fostering provider–patient communication about the quality and credibility of online health information, since 75% of US online health information seekers do not regularly check the date and source of the information they find (Fox, 2006), and some of the data they find is of questionable quality (Wajli et al., 2004).

Quality Improvement Movement in Health Care

As part of the movement to overhaul the US healthcare system, public reporting of standards are viewed as essential drivers of quality. Recently, Schoen et al. (2006) described the development of a national scorecard system using national and international data spanning domains of health outcomes, quality, access, efficiency, and equity. These are the major attributes which, when addressed fully, are considered to characterize a high performance healthcare system (Kilbridge, 2002; The Commonwealth Fund Commission on a High Performance Health System, 2006). Several challenges exist to broadly implement such a rating system, including a reliance on healthcare organizations and provider groups to voluntarily report their outcomes; consensus on the appropriate measures and metrics for the range of disease and illness conditions; the need for incentives, both positive and negative, to encourage healthcare organizations and provider groups to adopt and deploy such systems; and engaging patients to become more aware of and utilize these rating systems in making their decisions about where to seek care. It is this latter challenge that may be influenced or addressed by eHealth programs, e.g., Web sites that promote these rating systems in a patient-friendly and useful manner.

Public Reporting Standards

To enhance quality in health care, a number of federal agencies and panels such as the Agency for Health Care Research and Quality and the US Preventive Services Task Force (Whitlock, 2002) as well as public associations including NCQA and the National Quality Forum have promulgated clinical standards and guidelines for evidence-based care across major diseases and illness conditions and recommended prevention services. As an example, the Adult Treatment Panel III (ATPIII) of the National Cholesterol Education Program recommended guidelines for cholesterol management to improve the rate of appropriate treatment for lipid disorders nationally (Grundy et al., 2004; Smith, Cox, & Bartell, 2006).

Eaton, Goldman, Parker, and Cover (2003) created an eHealth system to both prepare and activate patients, as well as provide evidence-based clinical decision support to primary care clinicians, for cholesterol screening and care according to the updated ATPIII guidelines (http://www.heartage.com). The goals were not only to improve the management of cholesterol within the primary care setting, but also to determine the most effective way to engage and activate ethnically and socioeconomically diverse patients to have an ongoing dialog with their providers about their cholesterol, thereby stimulating appropriate care based upon established risk profiles and the evidence-based guidelines. As part of a randomized controlled trial funded by the National Heart, Lung, and Blood Institute, Eaton et al. conducted a series of focus groups with diverse patients (low-income patients and Hispanics were included), and providers separately, to determine the nature and understanding that patients had about cholesterol and its importance to their health (Goldman et al., 2006; Parker et al., in press). Results indicated that patients were confused about the true nature and meaning of cholesterol and its critical importance to their health, notwithstanding all of the direct-to-consumer advertising and promotion by pharmaceutical manufacturers. Thus, the creation and use of evidence-based guidelines and reporting standards by healthcare professionals is not enough to engage patients in learning about and understanding the health issues that they are confronting. This is another point at which eHealth applications may connect patients and consumers with the information and medical care that they need to achieve optimal health.

Emergence of Evidence-Based eHealth Applications

Mounting research evidence demonstrates the effectiveness of evidence-based interventions to help individuals reduce multiple risk behaviors, such as tobacco use or unhealthy diets, and to improve health-related behaviors, such as active coping, for chronic disease management (Goldstein, Whitlock, & DePue, 2004). Behavioral counseling by primary care providers to discontinue tobacco use, for example, significantly increases abstinence rates and is now the standard of care promulgated by the United States Preventive Services Task Force. A major barrier, however, to the impact and reach of these evidence-based prevention interventions can be attributed to the limitations of time and resources characteristic of today's busy primary care practices and health centers. Considering the numerous demands on primary care providers to deliver services for patients who are acutely or chronically ill, it is estimated that, on an average, there is only 1 min available for prevention activities during a routine office visit (Stange, Woolf, & Gjeltema, 2002). Although there are efforts underway to transform the primary care setting to become more amenable to behavioral risk factor prevention and chronic illness management (Glasgow et al., 2005; Rothman & Wagner, 2003), primary care providers presently have little capacity to deliver these evidence-based behavior change and disease management interventions efficiently.

Hence, quality of care suffers with respect to the use of recommended, evidenced-based prevention strategies.

Given this reality, patients are independently seeking out personally relevant health information and becoming more activated through the use of eHealth applications in their pursuit of better health and improved quality of life. Recent and ongoing changes in health insurance plans further reinforce and drive more consumer involvement and decision-making regarding the choice and use of healthcare providers and services. Consumer-driven health plans, for example, which shift greater financial risk and management to the consumer, are becoming more common as a way for employers to contain costs (Wilensky, 2006). The effect on quality with these types of plans, however, remains unclear, with recent evidence indicating a somewhat mixed picture (Buntin et al., 2006). This convergence of factors is likely to drive more investment in the development and deployment of increasingly sophisticated and personalized eHealth applications, as discussed below.

Consumer Role in Stimulating Growth of eHealth Applications

Concomitant with the development of effective interventions for behavior change and chronic disease management, consumers are increasingly using eHealth applications to seek health information for themselves or family and friends, to connect with others who have a similar disease or illness, and to communicate with healthcare providers. The use of the Internet for seeking health information, in particular, has become increasingly commonplace in the US. A survey conducted by the Pew Internet and American Life Project found that 79% (95 million people) of all adult Americans who use the Internet have searched online for health information (an increase from 50% just 2 years prior), making it one of the most popular online activities (after e-mail and researching a product or service before buying) (Fox, 2005; Fox & Fallows, 2003).

The increasing use of mobile wireless devices, such as cellular phones and Internet-enabled PDAs, creates opportunities for patients and providers to benefit from access to emerging eHealth applications for health behavior change and disease management in nontraditional settings (e.g., home, workplace). These technologies offer individuals the ability to obtain and utilize health information at relatively low cost, including people with limited access to healthcare professionals or services, and historically underserved populations. Healthcare organizations are using these technologies to improve the reach and efficacy of self-management programs and to enable enhanced communication between patients and providers. eHealth applications have emerged not only as potential vehicles for facilitating delivery of evidence-based care, but also as unique conduits to provide tailoring and customization based upon personal characteristics such as age, race, gender, ethnicity, sexual orientation, and primary language that would otherwise be unachievable and have shown to be effective in behavior change and disease management (Etter, 2005; Rothert et al., 2006; Vandelanotte, De Bourdeandhuij, Sallis, Spittaels,

& Brug, 2005; Wise et al. 2006). In addition, eHealth applications, if effective, have tremendous capacity for scalability at a potentially lower cost than what currently exists in our fragmented healthcare system.

Barriers to adoption of these technologies exist, however, including limitations of access, health and technology literacy, quality, and cost (Chang et al., 2004). There is also a legitimate concern about the quality of health information available through the Internet (Fox, 2006; Wajli et al., 2004), although increasingly patients believe they are able to assess the quality of the information, or can vet the information with their healthcare clinicians. Nevertheless, these challenges of quality and access, as noted above, must be addressed in order to realize the full potential of eHealth to support patient engagement for behavior change and disease management.

eHealth Tools

Below is a description of some eHealth tools that have the potential to engage consumers more extensively in the management of their own health care.

Provider–Patient Electronic Communication and eVisits

One of the fastest growing areas of eHealth is the use of electronic messaging with evidence that patients strongly desire to e-mail their physicians (Sands, 2000; Sittig, King, & Hazlehurst, 2001). Adler reported that over 47% of respondents in a study practice of approximately 2,400 active patients were willing to pay US$10 per year for online access to their healthcare provider or medical record (Adler, 2006). Another study found that more than half of those surveyed also indicated that the ability to communicate with their physicians online would have an effect on their choice of doctors and health plans (Harris Interactive, 2006b).

The content of electronic communications between patients and their clinicians varies greatly from scheduling appointments and requesting prescription renewals to caring for medical concerns that are not urgent in nature. The latter of these tasks, often referred to as an eVisit, has shown early promising results in chronic disease management (Patt, Houston, Jenckes, Sands, & Ford, 2003), as well as satisfaction among patients and physicians; reductions in cost of care, office visits, and telephone calls to clinicians; and fewer missed days of work for patients (*The RelayHealth webVisit Study: Final report*, 2003). Other benefits of eVisits and online consultations (which may be with a patient's physician or via online consulting services) for nonurgent issues included convenience and the ability to discuss embarrassing concerns totally or somewhat anonymously (Umefjord, Petersson, & Hamberg, 2003). However, when electronic communication is used to deal with care problems that are more complex, like mental health concerns, some of these benefits are lost (Moody, 2003).

Electronic Medical Record (EMR)

EMRs are generally housed within a physician practice, clinic, hospital, or integrated delivery system. Basic functionalities usually include documenting patient problems, clinical interventions, lab/test results, and prescribed medications (Kilbridge, 2002), essentially automating what had been previously located in paper records, though sometimes without clarity about the objectives of this computerization (Elberg, 2001). Though there has been limited research done to date to assess the impact of providing patients some access to their EMRs, one study found that log-on rates varied greatly, with most patients primarily being interested in lab results (Cimino, Patel, & Kushniruk, 2002). However, both patients and providers agreed that an EMR link improved provider–patient communications. In a recent study, Adler reported that patients were most interested in functions of an EMR that provided, in order, e-mail access to their physicians, the ability to review certain aspects of their medical records, and the ability to obtain prescription medication refills (Adler, 2006).

While the implementation of EMR-based systems faces significant challenges such as cost, lack of standards, limited patient input, low levels of interoperability between organizations, integration and portability, there is mounting evidence that the use of EMRs has the potential to improve efficiency, reduce medical errors, enhance quality, and positively impact patient service (Bates, Ebell, Gotlieb, Zapp, & Mullins, 2003; Grimson, 2001; Lesnick, 2003; Rotich et al., 2003).

A Harris Interactive/Wall Street Journal survey found that, given the choice, more than half of US adults would choose a doctor who uses EMRs and other technologies over one who does not (Harris Interactive, 2006b) Therefore, patients can play an important role in advancing the adoption and use of EMRs by providers and hospital systems in a number of ways. First, when selecting a provider or provider system, patients ought to include the availability of an EMR as one of the criteria for evaluating overall quality. Second, if a patient's provider does not use an EMR currently, he/she can ask why not and if/when the provider plans to implement an EMR system. Third, for those patients with health insurance, they can contact their health insurer and let them know how important it is for providers to have an EMR system to improve safety and quality. For many providers, particularly smaller groups, the initial capital investment required to install an EMR is cost prohibitive. In this case, as demonstrated in some regions of the US, health insurers have subsidized or offset some of the costs for computer equipment and software to establish an electronic platform to support an EMR.

Personal Health Record (PHR)

There is a growing consensus regarding the importance and value of the PHR as part of improving the health information infrastructure and supporting patient empowerment and self-management (*Connecting for Health: The Personal Health Working*

Group Final Report, 2003; Iakovidis, 1998; Sands, Tang, Sittig, & Christopherson, 2003; Ueckert, Goerz, Ataian, Tessmann, & Prokosch, 2003). Unlike institutionally controlled EMRs, consumers control information in and access to data within their PHR. Conceptually, the PHR is not linked to a single provider or health plan, but rather spans a person's lifetime, and can contain data entered by patients that might not normally be a part of an EMR (e.g., nonprescription medications and supplements taken by patients, alternative and complementary modalities of care). However, there are serious concerns about patients' willingness to use a PHR, particularly one offered by a health insurer (Sittig, Blackford, & Hazlehurst, 1999). Trust and concern about confidentiality and security appear to be the major factors which contribute to this reluctance.

At this early stage of development, many PHRs are limited in functionality and continue to raise questions about access to them, especially in emergencies (Kim & Johnson, 2002; Sittig, 2002). Additionally, as noted above, most healthcare providers do not have their medical records stored in an electronic, interoperable format or EMR, which limits the transfer of data from that source to an individual's PHR. Nevertheless, results from the report of the Personal Health Working Group as part of the Markle Foundation's Connecting for Health Initiative indicated that over 70% of respondents from a US household survey would use one or more features of a PHR: e-mail their doctor, track immunizations, note mistakes in their record, transfer information to new providers, and get and track test results (*Connecting for Health – A Public–Private Collaborative*, 2003). In The Netherlands, efforts are underway to create and support PHRs on a nation-wide basis (Beun, 2003).

With regard to enhancing quality, especially for disadvantaged populations, PHRs hold promise for enabling consistency of care, electronic access to information on health conditions, and enhanced communication with primary care providers (Baur & Kanaan, 2006). One compelling example of the reach and benefit of PHRs to underserved groups is the MiVia Program (http://www.mivia.org). This service provides migrant workers and their families in Sonoma Valley, California, with electronic health records via the Internet. Implemented as part of an overall program and effort to provide health insurance coverage and more coordinated health care to indigent workers, the program includes a portable personal emergency card and access to a password protected and secure Web portal which enables these individuals and family members to share information with medical providers and to maintain a continuity of care record wherever they go. By supporting and maintaining ongoing access to primary care, this system helps to reduce unnecessary use of emergency rooms and acute care services, as well as providing a sense of empowerment for these individuals and their families.

Interactive Health Promotion and Disease Management Programs

The eHealth movement has lead to a surge in the development of interactive programs and applications to assist individuals in changing their health behaviors (e.g., exercise and weight management, smoking cessation, nutrition, alcohol and other drug use) or managing chronic diseases (e.g., diabetes, asthma, heart disease). These interventions can be delivered via CD-ROMs, wireless networks, the Internet, or stand-alone devices that connect to telephone lines, and may include components as vastly different as biometric monitoring, health risk appraisals, electronic communications with providers, information provision, and list servs. Studies on these and other interactive eHealth applications note encouraging trends in behavior change or support the deployment of Web-based tailored interventions (Baranowski et al., 2003; Glasgow, Boles, McKay, Feil, & Barrera, 2003; Gustafson et al., 2002; Lenert et al., 2003; Lorig, Ritter, Laurent, & Plant, 2006; Oenema, Brug, & Lechner, 2001), but they also highlight such difficulties as lack of generalizability to diverse populations or health/disease states, maintaining participant enrollment in programs and sustaining changes over time, as well as integrating these systems into office workflow and showing returns on investment (Baker, 2002). There is some emerging evidence which indicates that remote disease monitoring has been shown to be a cost-effective component of disease management programs (Chase et al., 2003; Field & Grigsby, 2002; Liss, Glueckauf, & Ecklund-Johnson, 2002), and that patient-centered care can be enhanced with an electronic shared decision-making system (Ruland, White, Stevens, Fanciullo, & Khilani, 2003). However, because these interventions are in a nascent stage of evolution, no single standard or approach stands alone as best of breed (Briggs, 2003).

Nevertheless, such interactive and tailored programs hold promise for engaging consumers in recommended preventive services and disease management programs. As one example, Rothert et al. (2006) demonstrated the positive impact of an online, tailored weight management program offered to members of a large, health maintenance organization. Patients who enrolled in a randomized controlled trial and used the program Balance®, lost an average of 8 lbs over a 12-month period as compared to a control group that lost an average of 5 lbs. A key element to this program, and other similar ones is the tailoring on demographic, cultural, and social/behavioral characteristics, including readiness to change.

Patient–Provider Internet Portals

There is clear and convincing evidence, including ongoing demonstration projects by health plans, that leading health insurers recognize that members want more communication with their providers and seek contact with them using a secure Internet or "Web" portal (Baldwin, 2002; Slater & Zimmerman, 2002). For example, patients desire e-mail, eScheduling, eVisits, and ePrescribing with their clinicians (Chase et al., 2003; Sittig, King, & Hazlehurst, 2000). More and more, managed care organizations, health plans, and governmental agencies see value in offering these Internet-based services as a way to respond to growing consumer demand, to contain costs, enhance efficiency, and obtain market distinction in reaction to increasing competition (Kenny, Kongstvedt, & Shaman, 2002; O'Dell

& Hansen, 2003). For health plans that desire to be the primary and dominant health Web portal for members seeking health information, members expect and desire useful, reliable, and credible information from these sites (Ault, 2002). It is noteworthy that, presently, most people covered by private health insurance in the US look to mass-market Internet sites for health information more often than their health plan's Web site (Von Knoop, Lovich, Silverstein, & Tutty, 2003). That fact notwithstanding, at least 20% of households with coverage have logged on to their health plan's Web site, compelling these plans to meet members' expectations, including the challenges of maintaining data continuity with other administrative service channels (e.g., phone- and paper-based), as well as integrating and ensuring the quality of subcontracted services and links, such as health-related Web sites and disease management programs (Boehm, Holmes, & Yuen, 2003).

Examples of Patient eHealth Applications for Quality Improvement

Despite the relatively short period of time for eHealth to produce programs of high quality, a number of eHealth interventions have emerged which meet the criteria of evidence-based, developed with extensive end-user input, accessible to and tested with diverse populations, and are of demonstrated quality. These "best-of-breed applications" include such programs as QuitNet (Cobb, Graham, Bock, Papandonatos, & Abrams, 2005), Comprehensive Health Enhancement Support System (CHESS) (Gustafson et al., 2002), Balance (Rothert et al., 2006), HeartAge (Eaton et al., 2003), and MyHealthe-Vet (*My HealtheVet*, 2006, United States Department of Veteran's Affairs, 2006). CHESS, developed by Dr. David Gustafson, a pioneer in eHealth, provides tailored support and health information resources to diverse patients with breast cancer. Gustafson continues to explore and evaluate the impact of using the Internet to reach socioeconomically and ethnically diverse groups of women with breast cancer in order to provide support and various forms of tailored health information.

Another example is a project funded by the Robert Wood Johnson Foundation and housed at the University of North Carolina, Chapel Hill, to evaluate online support groups or "list servs" for various forms of cancer. The virtual communities of the Association of Cancer Online Resources (ACOR) afford participants a chance to interact with others, often anonymously, from across the street or on the other side of the world. ACOR offers a host of services to users including information and advice about medications, treatment options, and clinical trials; emotional support and empathy from those living with the same type of cancer; and practical tips for coping with symptoms. Individuals who are actively involved in ACOR groups may offer testimonials about the benefits of participation in them, but little research has been done to understand the components of what lists servs, in general, offer and how they may be of assistance to, or generate unintentional negative consequences for, their members.

To that end, Dr. Barbara Rimer is researching these virtual groups to answer this question: What is the impact on patients who participate in list servs? Rimer and her colleagues are conducting a 36-month, multimethod evaluation that focuses on the nature of the interactions that occur between participants in nine ACOR list servs.

Results of this study will have a twofold effect in the field of eHealth research. The first is the lessons being learned regarding the challenges and obstacles to overcome when doing research on technological interventions with real people in real time, many of whom are anonymous, and all of whom are grappling with a life-threatening condition. Because of this, traditional methods of communicating with study participants, gaining informed consent, and gathering data must be rethought (Bowling et al., 2006). Second, the results of this study will have significant ramifications not only within the field of cancer, but also across all chronic diseases. If beneficial patient outcomes (better quality of life, enhanced symptom management, improved patient–provider communication, etc.) can be linked to specific aspects of list serv interactions, virtual communities for cancer and other chronic conditions could be structured or modified to include these components. Under these circumstances, list servs eventually may hold the promise of minimizing pain and suffering for millions of people at little or no cost.

Future Directions for eHealth, Consumer Engagement and Quality Improvement

What role can eHealth play in the future to engage consumers for quality improvement? It has been our contention in this focused review that eHealth does and can help patients to better manage chronic diseases, and influence preventive actions and support self-care. However, while eHealth's potential to enhance behavior change and chronic disease management is promising, and the ability of eHealth programs to engage diverse consumers is apparent, the answers to these questions are complex and depend upon a variety of different factors, many of which were noted above, but warrant additional discussion and comment. Some of these are delineated below.

Health, Language, and Technological Literacy

Consumers and patients face a set of barriers in the use of eHealth interventions that could engage them in recommended prevention and disease management strategies, thereby improving their quality of care. Health and language literacy are salient throughout the healthcare system but can be doubly burdensome in the field of eHealth for patients who speak and read little or no English or who may have a reduced capacity to understand health information due to lower reading skills. For example, Web sites and other eHealth programs often assume a level of English language comprehension amongst their users that may not be achievable by those seeking to interact with these applications. In addition, individuals' experiences and comfort levels with using technology vary greatly and can have an enormous impact upon whether or not eHealth devices and applications would be used when made accessible. eHealth developers and those organizations that seek to employ these products must be cognizant of these challenges when designing technologically based interventions, test (and possibly modify) them with target populations, as well as providing end-users with appropriate training to use them.

Access for Traditionally Underserved Populations

Cost and usability are two challenges that people of color, elders, persons with disabilities, rural populations, low-income families, and others may confront in gaining access to eHealth applications. If interfaces (e.g., computerized devices) and the supporting connectivity (e.g., wireless technologies, broadband) are too expensive, or not designed with consideration to obstacles that some end users may face (e.g., those with visual or mobility impairments), this will exacerbate the digital divide and support a two-tiered system of those with eHealth access and those without. Some may argue that this will decrease over time as technology becomes ubiquitous and as aging, but technologically savvy, baby boomers make demands about eHealth access in the future. However, developers and researchers must not be complacent with respect to these challenges but rather focus attention on ways to mitigate or alleviate these impediments. Researchers need to be motivated by funders to make inquiries into this area of study a priority, especially in light of the Healthy People 2010 goals, which include the reduction of health disparities.

Cultural Relevance

The increasing diversity of the US population brings with it the reality that "one size fits all" does not work for eHealth programs. Different cultural patterns regarding concepts of health and health care, modes of communication, exercise and eating behaviors, and methods of seeking information will have a direct bearing on how, if at all, people choose to use eHealth solutions, even in the absence of language, technological, or access barriers. The development of eHealth interventions must continue to evolve and keep pace with the changing needs and desires of our multiethnic society. A strong argument for the commercial development of eHealth tools can be made here, given the nature of these changing demographics. There are many, as yet, untapped growth opportunities in this market. However, as with literacy issues, eHealth developers and others must maintain a keen sense of awareness around issues of design, testing, and modification of eHealth solutions for diverse populations.

Privacy and Security

Recent headlines have highlighted stories about breaches of privacy within consumer and patient information systems (United States Department of Veterans Affairs, 2006; United States Government Accountability Office, 2006). As a consequence, patients and healthcare providers alike share concerns regarding the confidentiality and security of Protected Health Information (PHI) stored in an electronic format. HIPAA security and privacy rules, encrypted Web sites, secure messaging, and electronic surveillance systems all play a role in reducing the risks of unintentional releases of PHI, but efforts must continue to strengthen the mechanisms by which PHI is safeguarded in eHealth applications, especially as the use of wireless technologies and other emerging tools (e.g., remote home sensors and monitoring) grows.

Interoperability, Infrastructure, and Integration

While many eHealth applications can achieve widespread adoption without a national infrastructure of interoperable EMRs, eHealth's full potential in the US is unlikely to be realized until this infrastructure is created and sustained as a necessary step to strengthen effective communication among patients and the multiple providers that form a care team. Developers need to be motivated to create and work with a range of technologies and systems which are interoperable with one another, as opposed to the many current stand-alone applications that only work on platforms within one health system or are available on one Web site. Integration of eHealth functions that consumers want and that respond to the needs of physicians and other health professionals will be key to moving adoption forward. More broadly, it is possible to envision a future where face-to-face and eHealth modes of prevention, disease management and monitoring, and care giving by both healthcare professionals and lay people are seamlessly integrated. This could enhance communication among consumers, patients, their families, and providers, potentially improving health outcomes and quality of life for all. Informed consumerism through eHealth will improve and ensure quality.

Conclusions

In this chapter, we present evidence to support the contention that eHealth currently, and in the future, will play a major role in engaging consumers and patients to become more involved in improving the quality of health care they receive for themselves and their families, as well as for the healthcare system as a whole. These predicted outcomes will be attained through eHealth's ability to help diverse consumers and patients to become more informed and knowledgeable about their health, activated in addressing their health concerns with their providers, and skilled in self-management. In essence, eHealth will enable and support the call for development of a more patient-centric, high-quality healthcare system.

References

ABC News/USA TODAY/Kaiser Family Foundation health care poll. (2006). *USA Today*.

Adler, K. (2006). Web portals in primary care: An evaluation of patient readiness and willingness to pay for online services. *Journal of Medical Internet Research, 8*(4), e26.

Agency for Healthcare Research and Quality. (2005). *National Healthcare Disparities Report, 2005* (p. 188). Rockville, MD: Agency for Healthcare Research and Quality.

Anderson, G. F., Frogner, B. K., Johns, R. A., & Reinhardt, U. E. (2006). Health care spending and use of information technology in OECD countries. *Health Affairs, 25*(3), 819–831.

Asch, S. M., Kerr, E. A., Keesey, J., Adams, J. L., Setodji, C. M., Malik, S., et al. (2006). Who is at greatest risk for receiving poor-quality health care? *The New England Journal of Medicine, 354*(11), 1147–1156.

Ault, A. (2002). Health web site users find information credible, but want content regulated. *Reuters Medical News*.

Baker, G. B. (2002). Integrating technology and disease management – The challenges. *Healthplan Magazine, 43*(5), 60–62, 64–66.

Baldwin, F. (2002). The doctor is in with physician–patient messaging, via web portals everyone is better served. *Healthcare Informatics, 10*, 44–48.

Baranowski, T., Baranowski, J., Cullen, K. W., Marsh, T., Islam, N., Zakeri, I., et al. (2003). Squire's quest!: Dietary outcome evaluation of a multimedia game. *American Journal of Preventive Medicine, 24*(1), 52–61.

Bates, D., Ebell, M., Gotlieb, E., Zapp, J., & Mullins, H. C. (2003). A proposal for electronic medical records in U.S. primary care. *Journal of the American Medical Informatics Association, 10*(1), 1–10.

Baur, C., & Kanaan, S. (2006). *Expanding the reach and impact of consumer e-Health tools*. Rockville, MD: US Department of Health and Human Services; The Office of Disease Prevention and Health Promotion (ODPHP).

Beun, J. (2003). Electronic healthcare record: A way to empower the patient. *International Journal of Medical Informatics, 69*(2–3), 191–196.

Boehm, E. W., Holmes, B. J., & Yuen, E. H. (2003). How to fix health plan member service: Part one. *Forrester Research*. www.forrester.com

Bowling, J. M., Rimer, B. K., Lyons, E. J., Golin, C. E., Frydman, G., & Ribisl, K. M. (2006). Methodologic challenges of eHealth research. *Evaluation and Program Planning, 29*(4), 390–396.

Briggs, B. (2003). The main event: Best-of-breed vs. single-source. *Health Data Management, 11*(6), 41–48.

Buntin, M., Damberg, C., Haviland, A., Kapur, K., Lurie, N., McDevitt, R., et al. (2006). Consumer-directed health care: Early evidence about effects on cost and quality. *Health Affairs, 25*(6), w516–w530.

Chang, B. L., Bakken, S., Brown, S., Houston, T. K., Kreps, G. L., Kukafka, R., et al. (2004). Bridging the digital divide: Reaching vulnerable populations. *Journal of the American Medical Informatics Association, 11*(6), 448–457.

Chase, H. P., Pearson, J. A., Wightman, C., Roberts, M., Oderberg, A. D., & Garg, S. K. (2003). Modem transmission of glucose values reduces the costs and need for clinic visits. *Diabetes Care, 26*(5), 1475–1479.

Cimino, J., Patel, V., & Kushniruk, A. (2002). The patient clinical information system (PatCIS): Technical solutions for and experience with giving patients access to their electronic medical records. *International Journal of Medical Informatics, 68,* 113–127.

Cobb, N., Graham, A., Bock, B., Papandonatos, G., & Abrams, D. (2005). Initial evaluation of a real-world Internet smoking cessation system. *Nicotine & Tobacco Research, 7*(2), 207–216.

Connecting for health – A public–private collaborative (pp. 1–7). (2003). New York: The Markle Foundation.

Connecting for health: The personal health working group final report (p. 55). (2003). New York: The Markle Foundation.

Eaton, C., Goldman, R., Parker, D., & Cover, R. (2003). HeartAge – A patient activation tool for cholesterol management. In: *Scientific proceeding of North American primary care research group, Banff, Alberta, Canada.*

Elberg, P. (2001). Electronic patient records and innovation in health care services. *International Journal of Medical Informatics, 64*(2–3), 201–205.

Eng, T. R. (2001). *The eHealth landscape: A terrain map of emerging information and communication technologies in health and health care* (pp. 1–137). Princeton, NJ: The Robert Wood Johnson Foundation.

Etter, J. (2005). Comparing the efficacy of two internet-based, computer-tailored smoking cessation programs: A randomized trial. *Journal of Medical Internet Research, 7*(1), e2.

Field, M., & Grigsby, J. (2002). Telemedicine and remote patient monitoring. *Journal of the American Medical Association, 288*(4), 423–425.

Fox, S. (2005). Health information online. Washington, DC: Pew Internet & American Life Project.

Fox, S. (2006). Online health search 2006: Most internet users start at a search engine when looking for health information online. Very few check the source and date of the information they find (p. 15). Washington, DC: Pew Internet & American Life Project.

Fox, S., & Fallows, D. (2003). Internet health resources: Health searches and email have become commonplace, but there is room for improvement in searches and overall Internet access (p. 35). Washington, DC: Pew Internet & American Life Project.

Glasgow, R. E., Boles, S. M., McKay, H. G., Feil, E. G., & Barrera, M. (2003). The D-Net diabetes self-management program: Long-term implementation, outcomes, and generalization results. *Preventive Medicine, 36*(4), 410–419.

Glasgow, R. E., Ory, M. G., Kleges, L. M., Cifuentes, M., Fernald, D. H., & Green, L. A. (2005). Practical and relevant self-report measures of patient health behaviors for primary care research. *Annals of Family Medicine, 3*(1), 73–81.

Goldman, R., Parker, D., Eaton, C., Borkan, J., Gramling, R., Cover, R., et al. (2006). Patients' perceptions of cholesterol, cardiovascular disease risk, and risk communication strategies. *Annals of Family Medicine, 4*(3), 205–212.

Goldstein, M. G., Whitlock, E., & DePue, J. (2004). Multiple health risk behavior interventions in primary care: Summary of research evidence. *American Journal of Preventive Medicine, 27*(Suppl. 1), 61–79.

Grimson, J. (2001). Delivering the electronic healthcare record for the 21st century. *International Journal of Medical Informatics, 64*(2–3), 111–127.

Grundy, S. M., Cleeman, J. I., Merz, C. N. B., Brewer, H. B., Clark, L. T., Hunninghake, D. B., et al. (2004). Implications of recent clinical trials for the National Cholesterol Education Program Adult Treatment Panel III Guidelines. *Circulation, 110,* 227–239.

Gustafson, D. H., Hawkins, R. P., Boberg, E. W., McTavish, F., Owens, B., Wise, M., et al. (2002). CHESS: 10 years of research and development in consumer health informatics for broad populations, including the underserved. *International Journal of Medical Informatics, 65,* 169–177.

Harris Interactive. (2005a). Public interest in the use of quality metrics in healthcare is mixed – Unless it allows them to reduce their health insurance costs (p. 6). Rochester, NY: Harris Interactive.

Harris Interactive. (2005b). Many nationwide believe in the potential benefits of electronic medical records and are interested in online communications with physicians (p. 5). Rochester, NY: Harris Interactive.

Harris Interactive. (2005c). New poll shows US adults strongly favor and value new medical technologies in their doctor's office (p. 6). Rochester, NY: Harris Interactive.

Harris Interactive. (2006a). Number of "Cyberchondriacs" – Adults who have ever gone online for health information – Increases to an estimated 136 million nationwide (p. 5). Rochester, NY: Harris Interactive.

Harris Interactive. (2006b). Few patients use or have access to online services for communicating with their doctors, but most would like to (p. 7). Rochester, NY: Harris Interactive.

Horrigan, J. B., & Rainie, L. (2002). Counting on the Internet: Most expect to find key information online; most find the information they seek; many now turn to the internet first (p. 17). Washington, DC: Pew Internet & American Life Project.

Iakovidis, I. (1998). Towards personal health record: Current situation, obstacles, and trends in implementation of electronic healthcare record in Europe. *International Journal of Medical Informatics, 52*, 105–115.

Kenny, S., Kongstvedt, P., & Shaman, H. (2002). *A survey of Payor web sites: How health plans are using the Internet to reach consumers* (p. 14). McLean, VA: Cap, Gemini, Ernst and Young.

Kilbridge, P. (2002). *Crossing the chasm with information technology: Bridging the quality gap in health care* (p. 32). Oakland, CA: California HealthCare Foundation.

Kim, M., & Johnson, K. (2002). Personal health records: Evaluation of functionality and utility. *Journal of the American Medical Informatics Association, 9*(2), 171–180.

Lenert, L., Munoz, R. F., Stoddard, J., Delucchi, K., Bansod, A., Skoczen, S., et al. (2003). Design and pilot evaluation of an internet smoking cessation program. *Journal of the American Medical Informatics Association, 10*, 16–20.

Lesnick, B. (2003). Taking it to the next level: Georgia specialty practice provides greater care by improving efficiency with EMR system. *Health Management Technology*. www.healthmgttech.com

Liss, H., Glueckauf, R., & Ecklund-Johnson, E. (2002). Research on telehealth and chronic medical conditions: Critical review, key issues, and future directions. *Rehabilitation Psychology, 47*(1), 8–30.

Liu, J. H., Zingmond, D. S., McGory, M. L., SooHoo, N. F., Ettner, S. L., Brook, R. H., et al. (2006). Disparities in the utilization of high-volume hospitals for complex surgery. *Journal of the American Medical Association, 296*(16), 1973–1980.

Lorig, K. R., Ritter, P. L., Laurent, D. D., & Plant, K. (2006). Internet-based chronic disease self-management: A randomized trial. *Medical Care, 44*(11), 964–971.

McGlynn, E., Asch, S., Adams, J., Keesey, J., Hicks, J., DeCristofaro, A., et al. (2003). The quality of health care delivered to adults in the United States. *The New England Journal of Medicine, 348*(26), 2635–3077.

Moody, R. (2003). Patient e-mails: Time pit or newest profit center? *The Business Journal of Portland*, e2.

My HealtheVet. (2006). United States Department of Veteran's Affairs.

National Committee for Quality Assurance. (2006). *The state of health care quality 2006* (p. 84). Washington, DC: National Committee for Quality Assurance.

O'Dell, S., & Hansen, J. (2003). The next-generation health plan: Not if, but when and how. *Healthplan, March–April*, 54–58.

Oenema, A., Brug, J., & Lechner, L. (2001). Web-based tailored nutrition education: Results of a randomized controlled trial. *Health Education Research, 16*(6), 647–660.

Parker, D. R., Gramling, R., Goldman, R. E., Eaton, C. B., Ahern, D. K., Cover, R. T., et al. (in press) Clinical practice guidelines: The complex journey from guideline dissemination to guideline adoption in the primary care setting. *Annals of Family Medicine*.

Patt, M., Houston, T. K., Jenckes, M. W., Sands, D. Z., & Ford, D. E. (2003). Doctors who are using e-mail with their patients: A qualitative exploration. *Journal of Medical Internet Research, 5*(2), e9.

Rothert, K., Strecher V. J., Doyle, L., Caplan, W., Joyce, J., Jimison, H., et al. (2006). Web-based weight management programs in an integrated health care setting: A randomized, controlled trial. *Obesity Research, 14*(2), 266–272.

Rothman, A. A., & Wagner, E. H. (2003). Chronic illness management: What is the role of primary care? *Annals of Internal Medicine, 138*(3), 256–261.

Rotich, J. K., Hannan, T. J., Smith, F. E., Bii, J., Odero, W. W., Vu, N., et al. (2003). Installing and implementing a computer-based patient record system in Sub-Saharan Africa: The Mosoriot Medical Record System. *Journal of the American Medical Informatics Association, 10*(4), 295–303.

Ruland, C., White, T., Stevens, M., Fanciullo, G., & Khilani, S. M. (2003). Effects of a computerized system to support shared decision making in symptom management of cancer patients: Preliminary results. *Journal of the American Medical Informatics Association, 10*(6), 573–579.

Sands, D. (2000). Using e-mail in clinical care: A practical approach combining the best of high tech and high touch. *The Informatics Review* (www.informatics-review.com/thoughts/patemail.html).

Sands, D., Tang, P., Sittig, D., & Christopherson, G. (2003). *Sharing electronic medical record information with patients via the internet* (p. 2). Boston: Medical Records Institute.

Schoen, C., Davis, K., How, S. K. H., & Schoenbaum, S. C. (2006) US health system performance: A national scorecard. *Health Affairs, 25*, w457–w475.

Sittig, D. F. (2002). Personal health records on the internet: A snapshot of the pioneers at the end of the 20th century. *International Journal of Medical Informatics, 65*(1), 1–6.

Sittig, D. F., Blackford, M., & Hazlehurst, B. (1999). Personalized health care record information on the web. In: *Quality Healthcare Information on the 'Net '99 Conference*.

Sittig, D. F., King, S., & Hazlehurst, B. (2000). Provider attitudes toward patient-related email. *The Informatics Review*. www.informatics-review.com/thoughts/provider-email.html

Sittig, D. F., King, S., & Hazlehurst, B. (2001). A survey of patient–provider e-mail communication: What do patients think? *International Journal of Medical Informatics, 61*(1), 71–80.

Slater, M. D., & Zimmerman, D. E. (2002). Characteristics of health-related web sites identified by common internet portals. *Journal of the American Medical Association, 288*(3), 316–317.

Smith, M., Cox, E., & Bartell, J. (2006). Overprescribing of lipid lowering agents. *Quality and Safety in Health Care, 15*, 251–257.

Stange, K. C., Woolf, S. H., & Gjeltema, K. (2002). One minute for prevention: The power of leveraging to fulfill promise of health behavior counseling. *American Journal of Preventive Medicine, 22*(4), 320–323.

Taylor, H. (2002). *4-Country survey finds most cyberchondriacs believe online health care information is trustworthy, easy to find and understand* (pp. 1–3). Rochester, NY: Harris Interactive.

The Commonwealth Fund Commission on a High Performance Health System. (2006). *Framework for a high performance health system for the United States* (p. 20). New York: The Commonwealth Fund.

The RelayHealth webVisit Study: Final report (p. 8). (2003). Emeryville, CA: RelayHealth Corporation.

Trivedi, A. N., Zaslavsky, A. M., Schneider, E. C., & Ayanian, J. Z. (2006). Relationship between quality of care and racial disparities in medicare health plans. *Journal of the American Medical Association, 296*(16), 1998–2004.

Ueckert, F., Goerz, M., Ataian, M., Tessmann, S., & Prokosch, H. (2003). Empowerment of patients and communication with health care professionals through an electronic health record. *International Journal of Medical Informatics, 70*(2–3), 99–108.

Umefjord, G., Petersson, G., & Hamberg. K. (2003). Reasons for consulting a doctor on the internet: Web survey of users of an Ask the Doctor Service. *Journal of Medical Internet Research, 5*(4).

United States Department of Veterans Affairs. (2006). *Department of Veterans Affairs Statement announcing the loss of veterans' personal information: May 22, 2006.* United States Department of Veterans Affairs.

United States Government Accountability Office. (2006). *Privacy: Domestic and offshore out-sourcing of personal information in medicare, medicaid, and TRICARE* (p. 35). Washington, DC: United States Government Accountability Office.

Vandelanotte, C., De Bourdeandhuij, I., Sallis, J. F., Spittaels, H., & Brug, J. (2005). Efficacy of sequential or simultaneous interactive computer-tailored interventions for increasing physical activity and decreasing fat intake. *Annals of Behavioral Medicine, 29*(2), 138–146.

Von Knoop, C., Lovich, D., Silverstein, M. B., & Tutty, M. (2003). *Vital signs e-Health in the United States* (pp. 1–40). Boston: The Boston Consulting Group.

Wajli, M., Sagaram, S., Sagaram, D., Meric-Bernstam, F., Johnson, C., Mirza, N. Q., et al. (2004). Efficacy of quality criteria to identify potentially harmful information: A cross-sectional survey of complementary and alternative medicine web sites. *Journal of Medical Internet Research, 6*(2), e21.

Wennberg, J. E., Fisher, E. S., Sharp, S. M., McAndrew, M., & Bronner, K. K. (2006). *The care of patients with severe chronic illness: An online report on the medicare program by the Dartmouth Atlas Project* (p. 108). Hanover, NH: Dartmouth Medical School, The Center for the Evaluative Clinical Sciences.

Whitlock, E. (2002). Evaluating primary care behavioral counseling interventions. *American Journal of Preventive Medicine, 22*(4), 267–284.

Wilensky, G. (2006). Consumer-driven health plans: Early evidence and potential impact on hospitals. *Health Affairs, 25*(1), 174–185.

Wise, M., Gustafson, D. H., Sorkness, C. A., Molfenter, T., Staresinic, A., Meis, T., et al. (2007). Internet telehealth for pediatric asthma case management: Integrating computerized and case manager features for tailoring a web-based asthma education program. *Health Promotion Practice, 8*(3), 282–291.

10
Medical Informatics

Rupa S. Valdez and Patricia Flately Brennan

Patient-focused information technologies, like clinician-focused information technologies are used to help improve patients' health. These technologies, which include electronic bulletin boards, patient-monitoring systems, and videophones, are used by patients, caregivers, and home-care providers to improve the health of patients outside the traditional clinical setting. Studies show that even with little attention to racial and ethnic factors, patient-focused information technologies may help reduce healthcare disparities between persons of varying races, ethnicities, and cultures. These disparities, however, may be further reduced through the use of culturally informed patient-centered information technologies. In this chapter, we discuss how patient-focused information technologies can be effectively designed to further mitigate disparities between racial, ethnic, and cultural groups.

Patient-Focused Information Technology

Patient-focused information technology, referred to in this chapter as patient-focused IT, is used to provide information, guide decision-making, and offer behavioral change and emotional and social support to users across boundaries of space and time (Gustafson et al., 2002; Moen, Gregory, & Brennan, 2007; Shaw et al., 2006). These technologies take many forms and serve diverse purposes. For example, by enabling patients to communicate with others suffering from similar conditions, electronic bulletin boards support behavioral change and offer social support. Personal health record systems enable patients to access, manage, and share their health information with others (Brennan, Downs, Casper, & Kossman, 2005), thereby providing information and guiding decision-making. A list of commonly used patient-centered information technologies and their functions can be found in Table 10.1. These technologies, which began as stand-alone systems, are now moving toward platforms such as wireless devices and virtual reality environments and have begun to include speech recognition and artificial intelligence technologies (Shaw et al.).

Table 10.1. Types and functions of patient-focused information technology

Electronic Information enables patients to readily find information about a particular concern. These technologies often link together multiple sources of information about a specific condition so that patients do not have to spend time searching for an answer to a question. Information may be presented as text or via another medium such as video. The primary functions of these technologies are to provide information to and guide decision-making of the patient and caregiver

Electronic Journals enable patients to record their thoughts, symptoms, and other experiences via a computerized application. The primary function of this technology is to provide emotional support for the patient

Electronic Bulletin Boards enable patients and caregivers to converse with others facing similar conditions via a computerized application. The primary functions of these technologies are to offer behavioral change and social support to the patient and caregiver

Personal Health Record Systems enable patients to access, manage, and share their personal health information via a computerized application. The primary functions of these technologies are to provide information for and guide decision-making of the patient

Patient Monitoring Systems enable patients to track their vital signs and other key indicators of health via a computerized application. Some patient monitoring systems are designed to automatically upload this information from peripheral apparatus such as a scale, glucometer, or sphygmomanometer, while others require patients to manually enter this data. The primary functions of these technologies are to provide information for and guide decision-making of the patient

Telehealth or Telemedicine Technologies enable patients and caregivers to communicate with healthcare providers at any time during the day. These technologies may be used in conjunction with other technologies such as patient monitoring systems to electronically relay information from the patient to a healthcare professional. They may also be used alone, as in the case of a videophone used to facilitate information exchange between a patient and a provider. The primary functions of these technologies are to guide decision-making of and to offer emotional support to the patient and caregiver

Videophone technologies enable patients to communicate visually with other patients or with caregivers. The primary function of this technology is to provide the patient with emotional and social support

As the name suggests, in contrast to clinician-focused information technologies, patient-focused IT is created for use by patients and their caregivers and not by medical practitioners. In this chapter, we use the term "caregivers" to refer to members of a patient's family or social network that care for a patient on a regular basis. The line between clinician- and patient-focused IT is sometimes gray, however, and at times clinicians such as home-care nurses use this technology with patients. For example, a home-care nurse may use a patient-focused IT such as a monitoring system with a patient. By discussing the data held in the monitoring system with a nurse, patients may be able to understand better the meaning of any trends in their vital signs. Similarly, conversation with the patient about data in the monitoring system may enable a nurse to understand better why particular patterns have occurred.

Patient-focused IT is intended to complement the usual care received by patients both in the clinic or hospital and at home following discharge. Under usual care, patients and caregivers must wait to communicate until visiting hours or communicate via telephone. Video technologies that enable patients in a medical facility to visually communicate with a caregiver that is at home, provide emotional and social support to the patient (Savenstedt, Brulin, & Sandman, 2003). Following discharge, usual care may consist of a home-care nurse checking in on a patient on a regular basis and providing the patient with printed information regarding their condition. Patient-focused IT complements usual care at home by enabling patients to access additional information regarding their condition electronically and to communicate with others who are suffering from similar conditions.

Patient-focused IT is further designed to increase a patient's control over their health care. Personal Health Record Systems, for example, enable patients to exercise more control over the care they receive in a clinic or hospital by ensuring that all attending healthcare providers have comprehensive and correct medical information. These systems may be especially beneficial when a patient is admitted into a medical facility such as an emergency department that does not have a complete record of the patient's medical history. The ability to search many sources using electronic information also increases a patient's control over their care.

Finally, although originally built for use at home, patient-focused IT may now be used in multiple environments. Stand-alone systems necessitated that patient-focused IT be used at home, where it was first installed. Web-based access to many patient-focused IT, however, has now allowed a patient to expand the place of technology use to the workplace, the library, and other public arenas.

Healthcare Disparities and Patient-Focused Information Technology

As discussed in earlier chapters, healthcare disparities are found across multiple lines including socioeconomic, geographical, gender, age, race, and ethnicity (Gibbons, 2005). These disparities are found in differences between environmental exposures, healthcare access, healthcare utilization, healthcare quality, health status, and health outcomes. Previously, patient-focused IT has shown promise in reducing healthcare disparities related to differences in access and utilization (Gustafson et al., 2002; Safran, 2003).

Many studies related to patient-focused IT have provided both Internet access and a computer to patients who did not have access to one or both of these technologies. The purpose of these studies was to gauge difference in utilization of the patient-focused IT in different populations in an environment where all persons had similar access to the intervention. These studies, therefore, cannot be used to assess if patient-focused IT would widen, narrow, or have no effect on access-related healthcare disparities.

A series of studies of the patient-focused IT Baby CareLink, however, does provide in-home access to all patients; therefore, the authors are able to draw some conclusions about the ability of persons living in rural areas and of low socioeconomic status to access the patient-focused IT Baby CareLink (Safran, 2003). Baby CareLink is a patient-focused IT that enables parents of premature infants to participate in decisions surrounding their baby's care even when they are not physically present in the Neonatal Intensive Care Unit. Safran found that approximately 300 parents of low socioeconomic status and residing in a rural setting used Baby CareLink more than 11,000 times during the course of 1 year. Parents accessed this technology from multiple locations including home, work, the library, and other public access points. These findings may be compared to a population of parents of low socioeconomic status residing in an urban environment who were given in-home access to Baby CareLink: Approximately 70 parents used Baby Care Link more than 600 times (Gray et al., 2000; Safran). Findings from these studies suggest that persons on the far side of socioeconomic and geographical disparities will not have difficulty accessing patient-focused IT and that they will actively use the technology.

A series of studies related to the patient-focused IT CHESS (The Comprehensive Health Enhancement Support System) found no differences in utilization across multiple lines (Gustafson et al., 2002). CHESS, originally developed in 1989 as a stand-alone system, is now an Internet-based patient-focused IT that includes services such as electronic information, electronic bulletin boards, patient monitoring systems, and an electronic journal. In a randomized trial of persons living with HIV, researchers found that there was little association between use and demographics such as age, gender, and race. Utilization was measured as the number of services used beyond a minimum time threshold and minutes of use within a service. In a study of breast cancer patients, it was found that underserved African-American women used CHESS as much as the more affluent majority. These results suggest that patient-focused IT may be effective in reducing healthcare disparities in utilization.

Patient-focused IT has shown potential in its ability to reduce access- and utilization-related healthcare disparities. Additional studies of patient-focused IT are currently underway to assess the impact of these technologies on disparities in health status and health outcomes. Given that patient-focused IT is still evolving, it is imperative that designers work to create technologies that serve the needs of persons who are currently on the disadvantaged side of the line. By doing so, it is probable that, like access and utilization healthcare disparities, outcome and status healthcare disparities will be reduced.

As stated earlier, patient-focused IT is not a substitute for, but a complement to, in-person care. Thus, although this chapter discusses ways in which patient-focused IT may be designed to reduce healthcare disparities, it should be noted that, to significantly reduce healthcare disparities, changes to in-person care are also necessary.

Cultural Factors to be Considered When Designing Patient-Focused IT

Although many factors such as gender, socioeconomic status, and age have been associated with healthcare disparities, the major determinant of differences is race and ethnicity (Smedley, Stith, & Nelson, 2003). Differences between races and ethnic groups remain even when income, insurance, age, and severity of condition have been accounted for (Graham, Guendelman, Leong, Hogan, & Dennison, 2006). For this reason, the remainder of this chapter focuses on ways in which future patient-focused IT can be designed to reduce healthcare disparities related to race and ethnicity.

Studies in multiple domains such as domestic violence, disaster management, and cancer screening have called for culturally informed interventions (Allen et al., 2003; Fernandez, 2006; Sumathipala, Siribaddana, & Perera, 2006; Taylor et al., 2006). Furthermore, studies have called for culturally informed interventions specifically as a way to reduce racial and ethnic healthcare disparities (Straits-Troster et al., 2006). This desire for culturally informed interventions stems from the recognition that there are underlying differences between cultures which, when attended to in the design of an intervention, are likely to make an intervention more effective than a generic intervention in minority groups.

Evidence of the effectiveness of culturally informed interventions has been shown in fields such as cancer screening and schizophrenia (Taylor et al., 2002; Weisman, Duarte, Koneru, & Wasserman, 2006). Taylor et al. found that by designing educational materials that were culturally accurate and sensitive they were able to, in comparison with a control group, increase the rate of screening for cervical cancer among Chinese women in North America. By attending to the cultural needs of both families of persons with schizophrenia and the patients themselves, Weisman et al. were able to overcome barriers to successful management of patients' diseases.

Because race and ethnicity are complex constructs, it is likely that there are many reasons for which disparities exist across their lines. Some may not be amenable to intervention; those that are include experiences with power differentials, mental models of illness, and language. After elaborating on these barriers to inequality between races and ethnicities, we offer a method of design, which when applied to patient-focused IT, may diminish this gap.

Experiences with Power Differentials

Power differentials between patients and the heathcare system may be especially uncomfortable for persons of minority racial and ethnic groups. Discomfort with this power difference is born out of historical reasons and is reinforced by current practices.

Both African-Americans and Native Americans have historical reasons for distrust of situations that contain power differentials. Race-based discriminatory practices against African-Americans such as legalized slavery and segregation as described in Jim Crow laws have led to a discomfort with these situations. Similarly, the confiscation of their homeland and other confrontations with the majority-run government of the United States has led Native Americans to be suspicious of situations that include power differentials.

African-Americans also have reasons for distrusting the healthcare system in particular. During the 40-year Tuskegee Syphilis experiment, African-American men in the end stages of syphilis were informed that they were being treated for "bad blood," when in fact they did not receive any treatment for their condition. Many died either directly from the disease or from complications of the disease. Furthermore, during years of slavery, African-Americans were used for medical experimentation. Many new medical and surgical treatments and techniques, including unanesthetized procedures were first tested on legally silenced slaves or freed Black patients (Dancy, Wilbur, Talashek, Bonner, & Barnes-Boyd, 2004).

Current realities also cause minority groups to distrust situations of unequal power. Relationships between minority communities and research institutes further enforce the belief that those with power are not to be trusted. Researchers often come into a community as outside experts, test their ideas, and then provide little feedback to improve the lives of the community members (Dancy et al., 2004). For this reason, members of minority communities often feel that they are being taken advantage of.

Distrust in situation containing power differentials is not confined to African-Americans and Native Americans. The healthcare system is also regarded with suspicion by other minority groups. In a study of attitudes of UK Muslim Indo-Asians toward transplantation, Alkhawari, Stimson, and Warrens (2005) found that many patients distrusted the healthcare system. Patients were afraid that by consenting to cadaveric donation, they might be prematurely declared dead so that their organs may be given to a White person. They further asked how they could be expected to trust the physician.

Negative experiences with power differentials are visible in many minority cultures such as the African-American, Native American, and Muslim Indo-Asian culture. While many such experiences took place in the past, several are still occurring today. These experiences, which took place both inside and outside the realm of health care, are a barrier to healthcare equality between races and ethnicities.

Mental Models of Illness

A mental model is a mental representation used to organize and make sense of knowledge, experiences, and observations about a particular phenomenon. Mental models about the nature of illness do not always transcend ethnic and racial boundaries. The majority population in the West believes in the use of allopathic medicine, or that disease can be treated by drugs that have an antagonistic effect to the disease. It is often taken for granted that all patients share this belief in allopathic medicine. Indeed the terms conventional medicine, standard medicine, and evidence-based medicine, which are often used as synonyms for allopathic medicine, underscore this belief that this is the "correct" way of viewing the health of an individual. Many studies, however, show that persons of minority racial or ethnic groups often have mental models of illness that do not include the philosophies of allopathic medicine.

Differences in beliefs about the nature of illness arise from multiple sources and have different manifestations. In the case of Native Americans, traditional views about health and healing are rooted in the race's philosophy about life, that all things are interconnected. Although each tribe has different belief systems, spiritual beliefs are important to all. For this reason, Native Americans maintain that a person cannot be healed without considering the spiritual aspect of their illness.

Belief systems about illness may also arise from experience. Communities that commonly experience a disease may understand the disease to be a normal part of life (Stanton, 2004). For example, a community that has recently migrated from an area where diarrhea or cough is ever-present may not feel that these symptoms are cause for medical intervention. Similarly, a community that experiences many manifestations of a disease may not believe that all of the conditions are the result of one underlying cause (Stanton). This may occur with diseases such as HIV that tend to manifest in with a wide array of signs and symptoms.

Finally, religious views may inform mental models of illness. In the study of attitudes toward transplantation in UK Muslims, Alkhawari et al. (2005) found that many individuals did not feel that it was their right to decide whether or not they would donate their organs. Instead, these individuals deferred their decision to religious scholars: If religious scholars interpreted the Qur'an as sanctioning organ donation, then they would consider donation. Furthermore, many of the participants in this study said that organ donation was not necessary and that if Allah wanted a person to live longer then they would live longer.

Although the dominant mental model of illness in the West is closely tied to allopathic medicine, many cultures do not share this mental model. Instead, mental models of illness vary between cultures and are informed by factors such as tradition, experiences, and religion. These differences between accepted models of mental illness remain another barrier to healthcare equality.

Language

A large proportion of the population who are on the far side of the "digital divide" do not speak English (Safran, 2003). In the United States, approximately 47 million persons do not speak English as their first language (US Census Bureau, 2003). Of these, 23% speak English "not well" or "not at all."

Translation is the primary means by which language barriers are often addressed. During translation, material presented in one language is rendered into another language. For patient-focused IT in the United States, this usually involves translating from English into another language such as Spanish or Chinese. Languages that are most spoken by persons speaking English "not well" or "not at all" include Spanish, Chinese, Vietnamese, Korean, Russian, and French (US Census Bureau, 2003). The goal of translation is to have a communication originally conveyed in one language have the same meaning when conveyed in another language. Barriers, however, to this process exist.

One barrier to this process is that the team developing the patient-centered IT does not include a person that is fluent in a language spoken by the target population.

In this case, the problem is a practical one. In other instances it may be possible to find a person that is fluent in both languages, but because of cultural values imbedded in language, it is not possible to directly translate the material from one language to another.

A study by McCabe, Morgan, Curley, Begay, and Gohdes (2005) found that cultural values imbedded in language prevented a direct translation between an informed consent form written in English into a written form in Navajo. First, because Navajo is not originally a written language, conveying the language by means of the Roman alphabet and phonetics was difficult. The vocabularies and grammar structures of English and Navajo also do not map directly to one another. This is the case for most pairs of languages, but especially true of languages that arose in the context of vastly different cultures. For this reason, the translation into Navajo from English often produced awkwardly worded sections. Finally, for underlying cultural reasons, entire sections of the consent form could not be adequately translated into Navajo. One section of the consent form in English stated that it would take each participant 40 min to complete the study. When translated into Navajo, this information was perceived as irrelevant because in the traditional Navajo context, time is not expressed in minutes on a clock.

Language can be a cause of healthcare disparities even among persons who are somewhat comfortable with the English language. Indeed, it can be a cause of health disparities even among persons whose primary language is English. This is possible for two reasons: First, persons who are comfortable speaking English may be illiterate (total inability to read and write), functionally illiterate (ability to read, write, and understand below the 5 grade level), or have a low level of literacy (ability to read, write, and understand between the 5 and 8 grade levels) (Cotugna & Vickery, 2003). Second, persons who are comfortable with everyday English may not be comfortable with written information on health-related items. Persons who fit this definition are said to not have health literacy, or the ability to obtain, interpret, and understand health information and use it to enhance health.

Significant proportions of persons of minority cultures do not speak, read, or write English well. Although translation has been one means of attempting to overcome this barrier to equality, obtaining an accurate translation can be difficult. Furthermore, persons who may have some degree of comfort with the English language may have some form of illiteracy. Thus, language is a third barrier to healthcare inequality.

Impact of Cultural Factors

If experiences with power differentials, mental models of illness, and language are not addressed in the design of a patient-focused IT, it is likely that persons of minority racial or ethnic groups will either fail to use a patient-focused IT or to misunderstand its content. For example, groups that have had negative experiences with power differentials are unlikely to use patient-focused IT; groups that do not have allopathic mental models of illness or who do not read, write, or speak English well may be open to using the technology, but are unlikely to understand its content.

This relationship between the degree to which the design of a patient-focused IT addresses (1) experiences with power differentials, mental models of illness, and language and (2) the use and understanding of a patient-focused IT is likely to affect healthcare disparities. If a community on the far side of the healthcare divide refuses to use a technology, disparities such as healthcare utilization may increase. Similarly, if multiple members of a racial or ethnic minority group act upon material that is poorly understood, disparities in health status and health outcomes could increase.

Fortunately, these relationships may also be harnessed to decrease healthcare disparities. For example, if experiences with power differentials are addressed during the design of patient-focused IT, any power-difference barriers to use may be reduced or eliminated. Similarly, if mental models of illness and language are attended to during the design of patient-focused IT, understanding of the content is likely to increase. This, in turn, may reduce healthcare disparities from utilization to outcomes. A graphical relationship of these factors is presented in Fig. 10.1.

As shown above, experiences with power differentials, mental models of illness, and language are all factors that define a minority racial or ethnic group. If these dimensions of race and ethnicity are not attended to during the design of a patient-focused IT, these technologies are unlikely to be used or likely to be misunderstood by groups on the far side of the health divide. Lack of understanding or use, in turn, may increase health disparities between racial and ethnic groups. Fortunately, each of these factors is amenable to intervention during the design process. The remainder of this chapter will describe strategies that can be used to effectively address each issue during the creation of a patient-focused IT. By attending to experiences with power differentials, mental models of illness, and language during the design of patient-focused IT, we can build upon the power of these technologies to further reduce healthcare disparities between racial and ethnic groups.

Designing Patient-Focused IT for Racial and Ethnic Minorities

Cultural beliefs and practices can influence the types and sources of health-related information desired by a community (Maliski, Connor, Fink, & Litwin, 2006). Consequently, cultural dimensions that are amenable to intervention such as experiences with power differentials, mental models of illness, and language should be attended to during the design of patient-focused IT. One method that can inform how these dimensions are addressed is user-centered design (UCD).

User-Centered Design

UCD is defined as a design and evaluation process that pays attention to the intended user, what they will do with the product, where they will use it, and what features they consider essential (Morales, Casper, & Brennan, 2007). For our

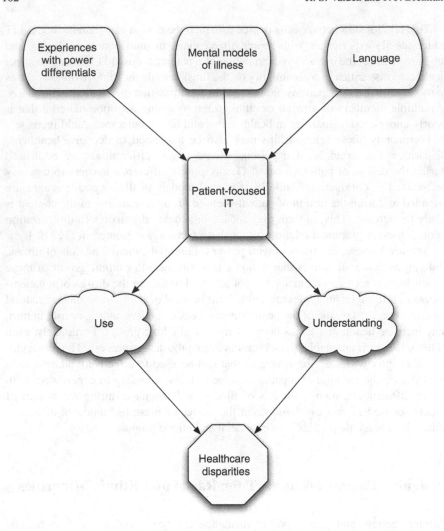

Fig. 10.1. Relationship between patient-focused IT and health disparities

purposes, UCD incorporates patients and caregivers that are the intended users of a patient-focused IT into its design and evaluation. In particular, UCD may be used by designers to address the concerns of racial and ethnic minorities about questions related to experiences with power differentials, mental models of illness, and language. Input and feedback obtained from users about these issues may then be used to inform the design of a patient-focused IT. Figure 10.2 provides a graphical illustration of the process of UCD in our case.

UCD has been shown to be effective in many fields. In aviation, this method was used to develop "cockpit navigation displays for low-visibility surface operations (Morales et al., 2007)." By taking the limitations and capabilities of the flight crew into account, navigation errors decreased by almost 100%. The adoption of UCD

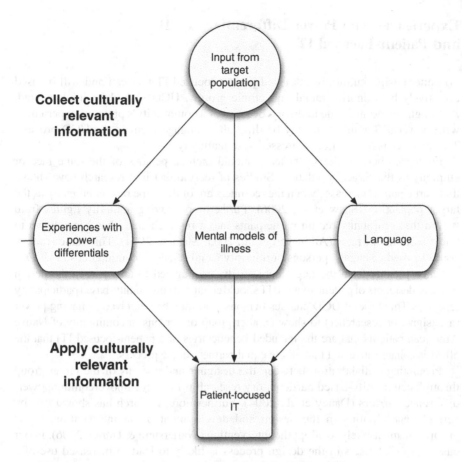

Fig. 10.2. User centered design for culturally-informed patient-focused IT

has also shown to be effective in the design of personal computers. When working on a redesign of the Think Pad, for example, IBM employed UCD. Users were asked to offer feedback about the current model and to offer input about ways in which improvements to the current design could be made. Results indicated that UCD was successful in increasing market share, brand equity, and customer satisfaction (Sawin, Yamazaki, & Kumaki, 2002).

UCD has also been effectively applied in the design of patient-focused IT. The patient-focused IT CHESS described earlier in this chapter used UCD in the design and evaluation of the initial intervention and all subsequent iterations (Shaw et al., 2006). Through needs assessment surveys, typically involving hundreds of patients and families, users were asked to check both the relevance and feedback of the content created by clinical experts (Gustafson et al., 2002). Although the impact of UCD was not tested directly, the high levels of utilization reported across racial, gender, and age lines suggest that UCD had a positive effect on the design of this patient-focused IT.

Experiences with Power Differentials, UCD, and Patient-Focused IT

To better design culturally informed patient-focused IT that can and will be used effectively by minority racial and ethnic groups, UCD should be implemented. Although this point is true in theory, because of a community's previous experiences with power differentials, it may be difficult to engage them in the UCD process. These power issues can be addressed systematically.

First, members of the UCD team should include persons of the same race or ethnicity as the target population. Studies of recruitment into research have shown that participation increases when the recruiters are of the same race or ethnicity as the target population (Shaw et al., 2006). Furthermore, having authority figures from within the community recruit participants into a research study has been shown to boost recruitment rates (Alkhawari et al., 2005; Stanton, 2004). This same strategy could be used to engage persons of minority racial of ethnic communities in UCD.

Once persons from the target community have agreed to take part in the design process, designers of patient-focused IT should engage in community-based participatory research. This type of UCD enables persons who may be perceived as having power (a designer or researcher) to show another group of persons (a community of Native American patients that are the intended beneficiaries of a patient-focused IT) that the effort is collaborative and that all are equal partners in the process.

Promoting collaboration between the designer and persons of the target group through community-based participatory research is effective in overcoming power-difference barriers (Dancy et al., 2004). Furthermore, research has shown that by actively participating in the design and development of an intervention, target groups are most likely to adopt the intervention (Wallerstein & Duran, 2006). In our case, involving users in the design process is likely to lead to increased use of a patient focused IT (Fig. 10.2), which, in turn, is likely to reduce healthcare disparities (Fig. 10.1).

Mental Models of Illness, UCD, and Patient-Focused IT

When a racial or ethnic group's mental models of illness differ from that of the designer's, group members are likely to have difficulty understanding the information presented in a patient-focused IT. Two approaches may be taken to improve understanding. First, members of the design team can teach members of the community about the mental model of illness commonly accepted by the majority culture. This may be accomplished though outreach presentations or other educational programs.

Although this approach is possible, it may be difficult or even impossible to change a community's mental model of illness, as many are deeply ingrained through tradition, experience, or religion. In this case, a designer's best option is to implement practices of UCD. Through community-based participatory research, for example, designers can work with members of the target population to fully understand perceptions about categorization of illness, severity, and vulnerability (Stanton, 2004). This understanding may be acquired by observing how the community addresses illness, experiencing traditional healing practices, and interacting with the community by taking part in conversations about health and illness.

Once designers understand the mental model of illness accepted by the community, they should take care to incorporate this knowledge into the design of a patient-focused IT. For example, if patient-focused IT is to be understood by some Native American tribes, it must include content related to spiritual well-being as well as physical well-being: A monitoring system could include ways to monitor spiritual health and personal health records could include a traditional practitioner's notes on the patient's spiritual health. Finally, any ideas such as the former that are developed by the designer should (1) be discussed with community members for assessment and (2) undergo usability testing, where users interact with a prototype of the final design. Any feedback obtained should then be used to further modify the patient-focused IT.

Language, UCD, and Patient-Focused IT

When a racial or ethnic group's primary means of communication is through a language other than English, translation of material originally written in English into a second language may be necessary. In this case, care should be taken to ensure that (1) the translation is adequately performed and (2) the translation is sensitive to differences in culture. To ensure the former, designers of patient-focused IT should find members of the target population who are comfortable with both languages. Often times, this may be a person of a younger generation who was simultaneously raised in both the minority and majority culture. One such community member should be asked to first translate the English version into the language of the target group. Another community member should then be asked to translate this version back into English. The adequacy of the translation can be measured by the degree to which the first and last documents match (McCabe et al., 2005).

Once this translation has been accomplished, designers should again review the translated documents with members of the target community. During this review, special attention should be paid to whether or not the translation is culturally understandable. If concerns are brought forth, designers should work with community members to revise the documents until the language used reflects group norms. For example, it may be technically possible to translate idioms such as "I feel downhearted and blue" from English into Gujarati, but this phrase would not carry the same meaning; in fact, it would be unintelligible. In Gujarati, the idiom used to describe depression translates into English as "I feel loose," a phrase that carries a very different meaning in English! These problems can be avoided by having users actively involved in the design process. After translation is complete, designers should use usability testing to ensure that the translated material is understandable and congruent with cultural beliefs.

Finally, designers' must also address language barriers that arise from varying levels of literacy. As in the case of mental models of illness, designers can implement outreach or other educational programs to bolster reading levels. Although this may be effective if the target population has a high degree of general literacy but needs help with health literacy, it would be extremely time consuming or impossible if the majority of the community is illiterate.

In these situations, designers must collaborate with users to develop innovative ways of harnessing the power of patient-focused IT. One potential solution is to have community members take part in the development of a video or voice over that conveys information originally in text format such as electronic information (Mandl, Kohane, & Brandt, 1998; Wood, Duffy, Morris, & Carnes, 2002). To ensure that the content presented is understandable and culturally and linguistically appropriate, persons acting in the videos should have the same ethnicity as members of the target community. Again, designers should conduct usability testing to ascertain the information presented in this format is understandable to community members.

Conclusion

Patient-focused information technology is an emerging field that has the potential to reduce healthcare disparities between gender, age, geographical, socioeconomic, racial, and ethnic groups. Some patient-focused IT such as Baby CareLink and CHESS have already shown that this technology may be harnessed to reduce healthcare disparities related to access and utilization. Other ongoing studies are currently examining the impact of patient-focused IT on disparities related to healthcare outcomes.

Even when factors such as socioeconomic status, age, and disease severity are accounted for, healthcare disparities between racial and ethnic groups remain. In fact, the largest gap between populations in terms of health care exists between these groups. Although there are many reasons for race- and ethnicity-related disparities, some causes such as experiences with power differentials, mental models of illness, and language may be amenable to intervention.

To help reduce healthcare disparities, designers of patient-focused IT should implement UCD to systematically address these three factors to create culturally informed interventions. Such interventions have shown to be effective in previous studies. Because each racial and ethnic community is unique, designers should work with each target community to design an appropriate intervention instead of trying to design a general version for all groups. When engaging intended users in the design process, particular attention should be given to dimensions that are amenable to intervention such as race and ethnicity such as experiences with power differentials, mental models of illness, and language.

References

Alkhawari, F. S., Stimson, G. L., & Warrens, A. N. (2005). Attitudes toward transplantation in U.K. Muslim Indo-Asians in West London. *American Journal of Transplantation, 5*, 1326–1331.

Allen, D. R., Carey, J. W., Manopaiboon, C., Jenkins, R. A., Uthaivoravit, W., Kilmarz, P. H., et al. (2003). Sexual health risks among young Thai women: Implications for HIV/STD prevention and contraception. *AIDS and Behavior, 7*(1), 9–21.

Brennan, P. F., Downs, S., Casper, G. R., & Kossman, S. (October 2005). *Personal health records systems: Essential elements and design considerations.* Paper presented at the meetings of the American Medical Informatics Association, Washington, DC.

Cotugna, N., & Vickery, C. E. (2003). Health literacy education and training: A student–professional collaboration. *Journal of the American Dietetic Association, 103*(7), 878–880.

Dancy, B. L., Wilbur, J., Talashek, M., Bonner, G., & Barnes-Boyd, C. (2004). Community-based research: Barriers to recruitment of African Americans. *Nursing Outlook, 52*, 234–40.

Fernandez, M. (2006). Cultural beliefs and domestic violence. *Annals of the New York Academy of Sciences, 1087*, 250–260.

Gibbons, M. C. (2005). A historical overview of health disparities and potential of ehealth solutions. *Journal of Medical Internet Research, 7*(5), e50.

Graham, G. N., Guendelman, M., Leong, B., Hogan, S., & Dennison, A. (2006). Impact of heart disease and quality of care on minority population in the United States. *Journal of the National Medical Association, 98*(10), 1579–1586.

Gray, J. E., Safran, C., Davis, R. B., Pompilio-Weitzner, G., Steward, J. E., Zaccagnini, L., et al. (2000). Baby carelink: Using the internet and telemedicine to improve care for high-risk infants. *Pediatrics, 106*(6), 1318–1324.

Gustafson, D. H., Hawkins, R. P., Boberg, E. W., McTavish, F., Owens, B., Wise, M., et al. (2002). CHESS: 10 years of research and development in consumer health informatics for broad populations, including the underserved. *International Journal of Medical Informatics, 65*, 169–177.

Maliski, S. L., Connor, S., Fink, A., & Litwin, M. S. (2006). Information desired and acquired by men with prostate cancer: Data from ethnic focus groups. *Health Education & Behavior, 33*(3), 393–409.

Mandl, K. D., Kohane, I. S., & Brandt, A. M. (1998). Electronic patient–physician communication: Problems and Promise. *Annals of Internal Medicine, 129*, 495–500.

McCabe, M., Morgan, F., Curley, H., Begay, R., & Gohdes, D. M. (2005). The informed consent process in a cross-cultural setting: Is the process achieving the intended results? *Ethnicity & Disease, 15*, 300–304.

Moen, A., Gregory, J., & Brennan, P. F. (2007). Cross-cultural factors necessary to enable design of flexible consumer health informatics systems (CHIS). *International Journal of Medical Informatics, 76*(Suppl. 1), 168–173.

Morales, M. R., Casper, G., & Brennan, P. F. (2007). Patient-centered design. *Journal of AHIMA, 78*(4), 44–46.

Safran, C. (2003). The collaborative edge: Patient empowerment for vulnerable populations. *International Journal of Medical Informatics, 69*, 185–190.

Savenstedt, S., Brulin, C., & Sandman, P. O. (2003). Family members' narrated experiences of communicating via video-phone with patients with dementia staying at a nursing home. *Journal of Telemedicine and Telecare, 9*(4), 216–220.

Sawin, D. A., Yamazaki, K., & Kumaki, A. (2002). Putting the "D" in UCD: User-centered design in the ThinkPad experience development. *International Journal of Human–Computer Interaction, 14*(3–4), 307–334.

Shaw, B., Gustafson, D. H., Hawkins, R., McTavish, F., McDowell, H., Pingree, S., et al. (2006). How underserved breast cancer patients use and benefit from ehealth programs: Implications for closing the digital divide. *American Behavioral Scientist, 49*, 823–834.

Smedley, B. D., Stith, A. Y., & Nelson, A. R. (2003). *Unequal treatment: Confronting racial and ethnic disparities in healthcare.* Washington, DC: The National Academy Press.

Stanton, B. F. (2004). Assessment of relevant cultural considerations is essential for the success of a vaccine. *Journal of Health, Population, and Nutrition, 22*(3), 286–292.

Straits-Troster, K. A., Kahwati, L. C., Kinsinger, L. S., Orelien, J., Burdick, M. B., & Yevich, S. J. (2006). Racial/ethnic difference in influenza vaccination in the veterans affairs healthcare system. *American Journal of Preventive Medicine, 31*(5), 375–382.

Sumathipala, A., Siribadana, S., & Perera, C. (2006). Management of dead bodies as a components of psychosocial interventions after the tsunami: A view from Sri Lanka. *International Review of Psychiatry, 18*(3), 249–257.

Taylor, K. L., Davis, J. L., III, Turner, R. O., Johnson, L., Schwartz, M. D., Kerner, J. F., et al. (2006). Educating African American men about the prostate cancer screening dilemma: A randomized intervention. *Cancer Epidemiology, Biomarkers & Prevention, 15*(11), 2179–2188.

Taylor, V. M., Hislop, T. G., Jackson, J. C., Tu, S., Tasui, Y., Schwartz, S. M., et al. (2002). A randomized controlled trial of interventions to promote cervical cancer screening among Chinese Women in North America. *Journal of the National Cancer Institute, 94*(9), 670–677.

US Census Bureau. (2003). *Language use and English-speaking ability: 2000.* Washington, DC: US Department of Commerce.

Wallerstein, N. B., & Duran, B. (2006). Using community-based participatory research to address health disparities. *Health Promotion Practice, 7*(3), 312–323.

Weisman, A., Duarte, E., Koneru, V., & Wasserman, S. (2006). The development of a culturally informed, family-focused treatment for schizophrenia. *Family Process, 45*(2), 171–186.

Wood, R. Y., Duffy, M. E., Morris, S. J., & Carnes, J. E. (2002). The effect of an educational intervention on promoting breast self-examination in older African American and Caucasian women. *Oncology Nursing Forum, 29*(7), 1081–1090.

11
Public Health Informatics

Bradford W. Hesse

Introduction

In 1973, program managers at the National Institutes of Health began working with scientists at the Centers for Disease Control and Prevention to assemble a network of data registries for monitoring the nation's progress in its newly announced "war on cancer." Data from the registries, the agencies reasoned, could be compiled into a commonly accessible database to track the incidence, mortality, stage, treatment, and survival of patients affected by the disease. Titled the Surveillance Epidemiology and End Results (SEER) system, this ambitious information system has provided epidemiologists and public health planners with the data needed to understand how the burden of cancer has been distributed across individuals throughout the population (Hankey, Ries, & Edwards, 1999). The SEER system has given epidemiologists insight into how environmental influences may affect incidence of the disease, and has provided health system researchers with the monitoring capabilities necessary to track efficacy of cancer control efforts (Edwards et al., 2005; Wingo et al., 2005).

After three decades of monitoring and analysis, population scientists using the national registry have at last been able to detect a reversal in the century-long trend of increasing cancer burden. Age-adjusted mortality rates attributable to cancer have been dropping steadily since the early 1990s, with substantive progress in areas such as lung cancer reflecting success in public health efforts aimed at controlling precipitants to the disease (e.g., exposure to tobacco smoke) (Hiatt & Rimer, 1999; Weir et al., 2003). In 2006, reports indicated the possibility of a first-ever decrease in the absolute number of cancer-related deaths (*Cancer facts and figures*, 2006).

Progress, however, has not been distributed equally. Analyzing trends from 1975 to 1999, SEER analysts have made some of the following observations (Singh & Miller, 2003):

- Socioeconomic differences in all-cancer mortality among men widened from 1975 to 1999. In 1975, the total male mortality attributable to cancer was only 2% greater in high-poverty areas than in low-poverty areas. In 1999, that difference expanded to 13%.
- Area socioeconomic differences in all-cancer mortality for women reversed from 1975 to 1999. In 1975, women in high-poverty areas experienced a mortality

rate that was 3% lower than women living in low-poverty areas. By 1999, that difference had flipped with women in high-poverty areas experiencing a mortality rate that was 3% greater than women living in low-poverty areas.
- The leading cause of cancer mortality in the US was lung cancer, attributable in most cases to exposure from tobacco smoke. Lung cancer mortality rates reached an all-time high in men in 1990 but due to the success of concerted public policy and public awareness campaigns it had a steady decline. Lung cancer mortality in women, who were targets of cigarette marketing later than men, continued to rise from 1975 to 1999.
- Socioeconomic differences accounted for increasingly larger differences in lung cancer mortality from 1975 to 1999. Compared to the rate of men living in low-poverty areas, the lung cancer mortality rate for men living in high-poverty areas was 7% greater in 1975 and 25% greater in 1999. Numerous studies have been initiated to evaluate the contributions of low socioeconomic environments on smoking.
- Mortality rates from cervical cancer, a disease that is largely preventable through routine screening, continued to show a strong correlation to socioeconomic status during the 1990s. Women in high-poverty areas experienced a 71% higher mortality rate from cervical canc er than women living in low-poverty areas.

Public Health Informatics

The cancer registry program illustrates what can be gained when a broad-scale informatics application is brought to bear on the problem of improving population health. Similarly extensive data collection programs have been established to monitor progress in the areas of nutrition (the National Health and Nutrition Evaluation Survey, NHANES), general health (National Health Interview Survey, NHIS), health behaviors (Behavioral Risk Factor Surveillance System, BRFSS), and disease outbreaks (Public Health Information Network, PHIN), to name just a few. As data from these systems are brought together to inform research and policy, they elevate understanding of health and illness from the individual level to the population.

Together the systems comprise the application area known as public health informatics, defined broadly as "*the systematic application of information and computer science and technology to public health practice, research, and learning*" (O'Carroll, 2003). The area of public health informatics holds the promise of documenting and diagnosing the pathways that lead to the unequal burden of disease in the US.

The Nature of Public Health

Public health is both distinct from and inextricably linked to the biomedical enterprise (O'Carroll, 2003). It is distinct in the sense that public health researchers have typically focused their attention on the health of populations, whereas biomedical researchers have focused their attention on the health of individuals. Historically, this separation of focus has given rise to slightly different perspectives on the population health problem, with public health professionals engaged proactively in prevention and health promotion efforts and medical professionals involved more reactively in diagnosis and treatment (Koo, O'Carroll, & LaVenture, 2001).

The tools available to the two fields have been historically different as well. Public health professionals use the social levers of policy and education to forestall problems at the macrolevel, while medical practitioners use advanced therapeutic techniques to intervene at the microcellular or structural level. Public health analysts must rely on data from surveillance systems, surveys, and registries to compile broad population-level views of outbreak and abatement; while biomedical researchers rely on data from physiological sensors to detect internal abnormalities and to monitor body system functioning (Koo et al., 2001; O'Carroll, 2003).

The two fields are linked in the sense that public health professionals work as partners with biomedical researchers to extend knowledge gained from the laboratory and the clinic into practice at a larger public health scale (Kass-Hout et al., 2007; Shortliffe & Sondik, 2006). Taking the knowledge gained from laboratory research on infectious disease agents into practice, for example, public health professionals worked with biomedical researchers to implement highly effective vaccination programs worldwide. During the twentieth century, this partnership all but eradicated diseases such as polio and smallpox, and created safer work and living environments through regulatory protections. Through dramatic advances in population health, this partnership illustrated how effective a combination of "science and political authority" can be in improving and extending quality of life (*Silent victories: The history and practice of public health in twentieth-century America*, 2006).

A Twenty-First Century Alliance

New views of population health suggest that the fields of biomedicine and public health will become even more closely intertwined in the next century (Mandl & Lee, 2002; Zerhouni, 2005). As argued by the director of the US National Institutes of Health, the victories of the twentieth century were accomplished with a biomedical science that was in its infancy; a science that used blunt instruments to attack problems of singular origin (Zerhouni). The battles of the twenty-first century, however, must be won against health threats that are larger scale, more complex, and formidable than targets in previous years. Chronic illnesses such as those associated with cancer, cardiovascular disease, neural degeneration, and obesity continue to take their place as the most frequent causes of death in the US.

Combating the seemingly intractable diseases that remain at the turn of the century will take a new armamentarium of biomedical and public health resources, an armamentarium built on scientific evidence and information technologies (Hesse, 2005). Whereas the health system of the twentieth century was reactive, treatment-focused, and oriented to the masses; the health system of the twenty-first century must become predictive, preemptive, and personalized to the needs of individuals (Culliton, 2006). A transdisciplinary, or "team science" approach, will be needed to tackle the most persistent health problems (Pestell, 2006; Sellers, Caporaso, Lapidus, Petersen, & Trent, 2006), including the pervasiveness of disparities in healthcare outcomes (Abrams, 2006).

A National Health Information Infrastructure

To win the public health battles of the twenty-first century, informaticians have argued for the necessity of tying together the nation's health information resources into a seamless network of tools, data, and people (Abrams, 1999; Buetow, 2005; Hesse, 2005). A seminal articulation of that vision was aptly captured in a report by the National Committee on Vital and Health Statistics delivered to the Secretary of the Department of Health and Human Services on November 15, 2001. The report, titled "Information for Health: A Strategy for Building the National Health Information Infrastructure," outlined a need for informatics development in at least three principal areas (National Center for Health Statistics, 2001).

The first two areas represented a reciprocal relationship between information encompassed within a *healthcare provider* sphere and a *personal health* domain. A key theme in these areas was the importance of developing a supportive informatics structure that allowed health records to be preserved electronically and transmitted seamlessly between healthcare systems. Such a structure would be impervious to disruption from natural catastrophe, with backups maintained in redundant and secure locations, and would allow patients to move between generalists and specialists or even between whole healthcare systems without falling victim to disruptions in healthcare support (Brailer, 2005). A protected infrastructure for records transmission would provide healthcare providers with complete access to a patient's medical history, even when patients have had a disrupted treatment history or an itinerant lifestyle (Chueh & Barnett, 1994). Safeguards could be built into the system to prevent medical errors, and clinical support tools could be built on top of the infrastructure to improve standard-of-care (James, 2005). Providing patients with access to their own health records would help promote a more proactive stance toward personal health and could help patients maximize their time between doctors' visits (Hesse & Schneiderman, in press; Safran, 2003).

The third area represented a macroview of data needed to protect *population health*, the area most directly related to the topic of this chapter. The goals set in this dimension included unifying public health surveillance architectures, streamlining quality and health status monitoring, and accelerating dissemination of evidence in order to preserve the health of individuals equitably across populations (Kass-Hout et al., 2007). Just as healthcare providers and consumers are interested in information at the individual level, the population health dimension was included to capture a planning need for viewing health data in the aggregate.

A spirit of shared overlap in the information managed within these three domains fits in well with the notion of a new alliance in the twenty-first century

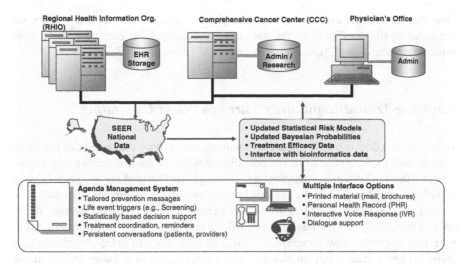

Fig. 11.1. Schematic illustrating how disease registry data from medical transactions stored redundantly within the office, hospital, and regional health information organization (RHIO) could be used to improve decisional accuracy through multiple interface options

medicine. In the bold new world envisioned by the report, naturally occurring data from electronic systems supporting the partnership of healthcare providers and consumers could be aggregated up (much as the SEER data are aggregated) to support population health decision-making. The aggregated data could in turn be used to update a biomedical understanding of disease etiology, and to refine the baseline considerations that undergird medical decision-making. This interconnected flow of data, collected electronically in clinical settings, synthesized and analyzed for public health, and then utilized in developing better tools for equitable health care, is depicted in Fig. 11.1.

Enabling a New Era of Research

Since the release of the 2001 report, discussions have expanded to include work being done in the area of basic biomedical research, a domain traditionally supported by specialists in bioinformatics. Enthusiasm in the area of bioinformatics has been catalyzed in recent years by success of the Human Genome Project, a project that made extensive use of distributed computing architectures to assemble data on the more than three billion base pairs comprising the human genome. Bioinformatics specialists are looking at the next phase of development given the massive amounts of data available from modern biomedical science and are turning to new informatics infrastructures that will help turn raw data into testable discoveries (Hesse, 2005). Whereas the emphasis in the previous decade was on new data collection and storage, the emphasis during this new era will be on "connecting the dots" within the data already collected, an emphasis some have referred to as an era of "Discovery Informatics" (Agresti, 2003).

Enabling Transdisciplinarity Through "Grid Computing"

To connect the dots in health research, bioinformaticians have suggested that scientists must be able to share data from virtually distributed work environments using a commonly shared informatics infrastructure. Although the World Wide Web represents a significant step forward in the area of knowledge sharing, computer scientists have noted that true data sharing has not yet been enabled through current Internet standards (Atkins, 2003). What has been needed is a new level of cyberinfrastructure support, one that will allow geographically distant colleagues to place compatible data elements into a shared informatics grid using agreed-upon ontologies and standards (Abbas, 2004). Once mounted onto this common, openly accessible framework, the data could be made discoverable to other researchers for integration into higher levels of analyses. Intelligent data-mining and visualization tools could be used to accelerate discovery across data sources, essentially shortening the time it takes to move from raw data to new concept formation (Burrage, Hood, & Ragan, 2006).

One instantiation of this new approach to informatics is reflected in the number of efforts investigating the feasibility of "grid computing." The notion of *grid computing* arose originally from scientists looking to take advantage of computing cycles among a distributed array of supercomputers. Much like the "power grid" balancing electricity demands among the various regions within a state, a distributed computer "grid" could offer load balancing in computational power as scientists set upon the task of analyzing vast amounts of data assembled simultaneously across an interconnected web of data repositories and real time sensors. The concept has been proposed by health scientists as a method for connecting disparate data resources into a seamless foundation for *en silica* modeling and discovery (Buetow, 2005).

Adding "Populomics" to the Grid

Admittedly, much of the original impetus for creating a grid of interoperable data systems in health can be traced back to the tsunami of isolated data streams emerging from laboratories specializing in "genomics" (studies based on the human genome) or "proteomics" (studies based on microarrays of biomarker proteins) research (Culliton, 2006). In the area of population health disparities, an equally compelling argument has been made to expand the national framework to accommodate data on the environmental and social influences that impact population outcomes, a field that has been referred to by some as "populomics" (Abrams, 2006; Gibbons, 2005). At the microcellular level, genomics and proteomics scientists are hard at work improving the predictive power of their risk models so that therapeutic interventions can be administered in a preemptive fashion to avert the onset of some diseases altogether, or to intervene in the earliest phases of disease when probability of therapeutic success is greatest. The same argument can, and must, be applied to intervention at the population level. At the macrolevel, "populomics" scientists must be at work identifying the specific pathways that lead to population health disparities, and must set out to update models of community risk to enable a more efficient application of targeted public health interventions applied preemptively, when the probability of success is greatest (Boslaugh, Kreuter, Nicholson, & Naleid, 2005; Broome & Loonsk, 2004; Fulcher & Kaukinen, 2004; Gibbons, 2006; Hiatt & Rimer, 1999).

As an illustration of populomics in action, scientists associated with the NIH-supported Centers for Population Health and Health Disparities, a series of eight large-scale centers grants awarded to teams of researchers to investigate multilevel solutions to the health disparities problem, have been collecting a broad spectrum of data to attack the health disparities problem from multiple levels of analysis. Investigations have been underway to assemble a framework for common measures across the centers that will be compatible with the agency's emphasis on data sharing, and that can serve to connect the activity to other initiatives through a common set of vocabularies. The measures under consideration span the range of analysis from microcellular indicators of genetic risk (e.g., BRCA1 risk for breast cancer), to biochemical assays of stress, psychological measures of coping, sociological measures of community, and architectural aspects of the built environment (OBSSR, 2006).

Enhancing Functionality in Public Health Informatics

Proponents of interoperable data systems argue that the time is right for the information revolution heralded by the first generation of Internet applications to evolve (Atkins, 2003; Buetow, 2005). Thanks to an extensive capital outlay in servers, routers, fiber optics, and high-speed cables during the 1990s, much of the basic foundation for a new generation of interconnected data systems already exists (Abbas, 2004). The entry of private sector powerhouses into the fields of eCommerce and eFinance has made online innovation a mission-critical activity in an increasingly more competitive and globally connected economy (Freidman, 2006). In many sectors, an advanced use of interconnected data systems has revolutionized the ways in which work is done.

Scientific disciplines have varied in their adoption of cyberinfrastructure capabilities, though. The ability of meteorologists to predict landfall of the devastating Hurricane Katrina in 2005 (an early warning accomplished through an advanced network of remote sensors, satellite imaging, and numerical modeling) stood in stark contrast to the collapse of infrastructure in delivering emergency services following the storm. The breakdown in information flow, severed along socioeconomic lines, bore an all-too-familiar resemblance to other breakdowns in public health infrastructure.

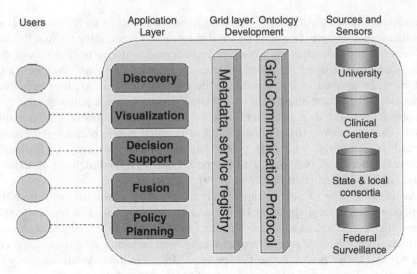

Fig. 11.2. A vision of enhanced functionality made possible by connecting public health informatics data sources through interoperable cyberinfrastructure

Strengthening the informatics infrastructure in population health is one step that can be taken to serve national interests in addressing disparate outcomes in health. Borrowing from the vision set by members of the Open Geographic Information Systems (GIS) consortium (Abbas, 2004), the remainder of this chapter presents a more specific blueprint for the expanded functionality that could be enabled by a connective infrastructure in public health. Figure 11.2 presents an overview of how the disparate system of data sources and sensors in public health could be brought together to enable a new level of application development. The functions filled by those applications are described below.

Discovery

The data being collected in the area of health and health care are plentiful (Safran et al., 2007). Large, national surveillance efforts collect sociodemographic and health information on Americans through the Departments of Health and Human Services, Labor, and Education. Local health agencies are regularly required to report vital statistics and incident data to state entities, and state entities are required to report those data to federal systems. Even the day-to-day administration of health care is becoming increasingly more data dependent, with hospitals and medical practices generating terabytes of data from laboratory analysis systems, pharmaceutical tracking systems, bioimaging systems, and administrative records. Federally funded research laboratories and community-based intervention efforts are generating constant streams of new, discoverable data each fiscal year. Arguably, the challenge confronting public health professionals is not in generating new data (though with new discovery, new data needs will become inevitable); it is figuring out how to connect the existing data streams into a usable framework in order to accelerate discovery.

In September 2006, the American Medical Informatics Association published a white paper on the topic of creating a national framework for the secondary use of health data. Reflecting on the input of a diverse set of stakeholders, authors of the paper highlighted the imperative public health value of using frontline clinical data to monitor for the emergent outbreak of a potentially contagious disease, or in improving quality of service universally across populations.

In order to reuse clinical data for discovery purposes, the authors of the report reasoned, administrators must build the privacy protections guaranteed by the Health Insurance Portability and Accountability Act of 1996 (HIPPA) into the management and electronic exchange of health information. To do this, administrators should (a) make policies on secondary use of health data transparent, (b) focus discussions on data control rather than ownership, (c) reach consensus on privacy policies and security, (d) increase public awareness, (e) build a comprehensive vision for data usage, and (f) seek out national (and state) leadership (Lumpkin, 2003; Safran et al., 2007).

Another aspect to the challenge of enabling discovery in the area of health disparities research lies in creating the structural coherence of a shared informatics environment. Much of public health data collection suffers from the same set of incongruities dogging biomedical research. Isolated data systems, balkanized knowledge bases, redundant reporting requirements, and disincentives for secondary data analysis are all too often the rule rather than the exception in public health (Jernigan, Davies, & Sim, 2003). Moving toward a shared information environment, as is being done within the Public Health Information Network (Broome & Loonsk, 2004), and agreeing on a common set of shared data standards, as being done within the Centers for Population Health and Health Disparities (OBSSR, 2006), is a necessary first step in enabling a evolutionary transformation of the science (Snee & McCormick, 2004).

Once a shared information space is enabled, tools can be built to accelerate discovery of the population pathways leading to disparities. Automated tools can be built to operate solely on data, and can be made to remove the subjective fac tors that often come from a purposive review of population data. Advanced data mining techniques, relying perhaps on the adaptive qualities of machine-learning algorithms, can shorten the task of discovery by sifting automatically through potentially generalizable patterns of data across localities. Integrating biologic data with environmental data will allow scientists to transcend the customary limitations of broad racial and ethnic categories, and to look analytically for novel patterns in gene by environment interactions (Strunk, Ford, & Taggart, 2002).

Visualization

One of the categories of tool development with great promise for researchers and decision makers investigating health disparity issues is the category of data visualization. Chief among these is the continued refinement of geographic information systems, which have migrated from large mainframe applications down to the desktop for individual analysts to use, and onto the Web for individual policy makers to use (Hanchette, 2003). GIS systems can be used to identify patterns of exposure as when levels of toxic exposure can be traced back to a commonly shared aquifer, or patterns of access as when geospatial analyses of late-stage cervical cancer can be used to identify areas ripe for community outreach to bring up levels of routine cervical cancer screening. They can be used by population scientists to investigate new relationships between the built and social environment on the one hand and health maintenance and disease on the other. They can be used by administrators to identify "knowledge gaps" (Freimuth, 1993; Viswanath et al., 2006) to focus communication efforts, and to locate resource gaps to focus budget allocation decisions. GIS capabilities were used by program administrators at the Centers for Disease Control and Prevention to portray the gradual progression of the national "obesity epidemic," with regional differences in eating patterns leading to more rapid increases in Body Mass Index.

As a cautionary note, because GIS systems can be very powerful in locating risk down to the individual address level, protections must be in place to protect the privacy of individuals. In one study, a full 87% of patients in a public use data set could be reidentified using zip code, date of birth, and gender alone. Most of the federal statistical agencies use suppression rules when reporting geographically identified data so that regional areas with $n < 5$ do not show up as distinct entities in tallies or maps. Informaticians can protect the anonymity of patients and survey participants by insisting that suppression rules and other techniques for deidentifying data be firmly in place (Cassa, Grannis, Overhage, & Mandl, 2006).

Other visualization techniques are being developed to promote insight in scientific discovery, to support decision-making, and to aid in the impact of persuasive or instructional messages. In the Human Computer Interaction Laboratories at the University of Maryland, computer scientists are developing a suite of interactive analytic tools that will allow researchers to select an individual data attribute onscreen, and then manipulate the data attribute to perform "what if" analyses instantaneously on-screen (Benderson & Schneiderman, 2003). As this work continues forward, it is easy to imagine how public health researchers might use these tools to identify the highest yield leverage points from the myriad factors contributing to unequal health outcomes. These visualization tools will be important to health disparities researchers as "macroscopes" of population trends (Litt, Tran, & Burke, 2002).

Decision Support

Surveillance data are collected with the express purpose of supporting public health decision-making. To that end, some of the national health and statistical agencies are experimenting with new tools to support evidence-based planning. One such tool, online at http://cancercontrolplanet.cancer.gov, provides state health officials with customizable access to data from the SEER registries described at the beginning of this chapter. Here, planners can specify a state and cancer site (e.g., lung and bronchus to track efficacy of tobacco control efforts) and then generate a county by county profile of incidence and mortality trends compared against national averages. Users can customize the profile to investigate trends by race/ethnicity, sex, and age, and can export the resulting values into a spreadsheet for further manipulation and planning. With customized data in-hand, state planners can use the site to obtain up-to-date prevention guidelines, find empirically tested intervention programs and products, and identify contacts for help in achieving objectives. This type of informatics support for decision-making should improve the success of individual programs by linking action to empirical evidence.

Medical decision-making is largely an inferential process of deducing the probability that a patient has a particular disease given the presence of certain signs and symptoms at diagnosis, and then selecting from a menu of treatment options to enhance the probability of success and minimize the probability of risk. Success in decision-making can be improved by updating the Bayesian parameters that go into the selection of tests or choice of treatment, either through decision aids or evidence-based guidelines documents. Informatics tools can be developed to support improved decision-making by updating decisional parameters through the use of real case, population data (Yasnoff & Miller, 2003).

On the flipside, the universal efficacy of clinical processes – and the informatics tools that support them – can be improved by aggregating data on those processes at a population level. This is the spirit of the series of reports generated by the Institute of Medicine's "Crossing the Quality Chasm" working group meetings (IOM Committee on Quality of Healthcare in America, 2001). To understand how medical care can be given safely and equitably across environments, members of the IOM working group compared the checks and balances in place within the healthcare sector with the processes in place in the aviation sector. Both sectors rely on complex systems and technologies, authors of the reports noted, but the aviation sector does a far superior job of protecting safety and quality universally for all those involved. The reason why, the authors surmised, is that the aviation sector has adopted a "culture of safety." It relies on a consistent stream of process data (near misses, sensor alerts, etc.) to create a self-correcting environment based on aggregate outcomes. Committing errors of judgment is a human frailty in both systems, only in the aviation system engineers have created the redundancies and supports necessary to compensate for errors upstream, before the errors turn into avoidably catastrophic outcomes. Efforts have been underway within the Agency for Healthcare Research and Quality to improve the universality of high-quality service throughout the healthcare sector (Clancy & Scully, 2003).

Fusion

The questions surrounding disparity in health outcomes are multitiered. To be effective, public health analysts must understand the etiology of population disparities across multiple levels: from the microcellular to the environmental, from "cells to society" (Abrams, 1999). The next generation of public health informatics applications should offer support for more extensive analyses of the conditions contributing to health disparities but giving analysts the ability to bridge analyses between sets of interconnected data. A comprehensive framework for cancer surveillance, to use one example, should span the entire life span and "be capable of providing information on risk, burden, disparity, cost, cancer care, survival, and death" (Howe et al., 2003). Plans for a National Health Information Infrastructure can make this fusion possible by encouraging the use of data standards, encouraging linkages through volunteerism and regulatory requirement, maintaining a fully documented metadata structure to place data within context, and by offering incentives to develop the statistical models needed to perform analyses across systems with dissimilar sampling frames (Chute, Cohn, & Campbell, 1998; Hiatt & Rimer, 1999; Jernigan et al., 2003; Snee & McCormick, 2004).

One of the most pragmatic reasons for motivating fusion technologies among currently disconnected data systems is cost. It has been estimated that by looking for ways to create interoperability between public health data systems, informaticians could save public health departments an estimated $195 million each year (Kass-Hout et al., 2007). Equally pragmatic is the urgency to save lives. After an outbreak of severe acute respiratory syndrome, or SARS, in Asia in February 2003, informaticians at the National Center for High-Performance Computing in Hsinchu, Taiwan leveraged existing grid projects to create fusion in a real time monitoring system between hospitals in Asia and the US Centers for Disease Control and Prevention (the CDC) in Atlanta. Creation of the Grid system, which was pulled together with only 2 weeks advance notice, was credited with saving at least two lives and extending the benefits of access from one of the leading public health agencies in the world to beneficiaries a half-world away (Ellisman et al., 2004).

The other, more content-driven, reason for working on methods to connect data systems is to enable an ability to move back and forth efficiently between levels of analysis. Many of the national surveillance mechanisms do a workable job at creating a broad view of health status across the national population. The broad view works well for creating descriptions of average trends, but lacks the sampling power to explore relationships within specific subpopulations. For this reason, the National Committee on Vital and Health Statistics has recommended complementing the general population samples with specialized samples into minority sample frames (National Committee in Vital and Health Statistics, 2005). The California Health Interview Survey (CHIS), as an example, collects extensive data on hard-to-reach populations of Asian-Americans, Pacific Islanders, and Native Americans. Efforts to bridge findings between the more narrowly scoped CHIS and the more broadly sampled National Health Interview Survey should allow researchers to transcend limitations from the broadly constrained sampling frame. Developing fusion technologies within GIS-enabled data systems, as another example, has been useful in helping resource planners consider multiple approaches to intervention, from broad communication approaches at the state to community-based interventions in localized areas (Fulcher & Kaukinen, 2004). Each level of analysis offers a different perspective on the disparities problem.

Policy Planning

A primary focus of public health informatics is to apply science and technology to the problem of preventing "disease and injury by altering the conditions or the environment that put populations of individuals at risk" (O'Carroll, 2003). For the most part, this means taking full advantage of the policy-setting levers available to public health practitioners to effect change in the environment. To make full use of the policy planning function in public health informatics, at least three conditions must be met. First, public health visionaries need to be sure that the science is in place to understand, predict, and control the conditions that lead to deleterious health outcomes. Second, government leaders need to ensure that the monitoring systems are in place to assess the impact of translational programs and environment-altering policy. Third, program administrators need to establish a strategic communication plan to be sure that findings from the informatics programs influence policy-making agendas in effective ways.

Regarding the first condition, congressional legislation has already called for the establishment of the National Center on Minority Health and Health Disparities at the National Institutes of Health, and a strategic plan to address the continuing poor health status of minorities, those with low income and people living in rural areas. In 2006, the Institute of Medicine released an assessment of the agency's strategic plan and identified areas of important, unfinished business. One of the prevailing themes, and indeed a theme reflected throughout this chapter, is the need for a transdisciplinary science to attack the problem of health disparities from a multidimensional perspective. That perspective would have to include an understanding of social, behavioral, and environmental causes in addition to an understanding of genetic and physiological contributors. The goal of implementing interoperability, by policy, among data systems is intended to create the infrastructure needed to bootstrap this new, integrative approach to disparities science. Along with connecting current data collection systems, program administrators should continue to look for gaps in the knowledge base, and call for selective sampling into populations that have been understudied (Committee on the review and assessment of the NIH's Strategic Research Plan and Budget to Reduce and Ultimately Eliminate Health Disparities, 2007).

Regarding the second condition, the National Committee on Vital and Health Statistics delivered another report to the Secretary of the Department of Health and Human Services on November 7, 2005 this time on the issue of eliminating health disparities. The report called specifically for strengthening data collection on race, ethnicity, and primary language in the US. To do this, the report recommended steps to (a) advance leadership, coordination, and partnerships; (b) increase availability of data on diverse subpopulations; (c) improve the collection of geography and socioeconomic position data; and (d) enhance data collection of disparities-relevant data through federal administrative programs, such as Medicaid. Efforts have been underway to implement many of the recommendations from the report, but work is still needed (National Committee in Vital and Health Statistics, 2005).

Realizing the third condition, that of implementing a strategic plan for communication, will take the sustained leadership of program directors working in close collaboration with informatics specialists. What is critical to recognize is that every interface intended to place informatics data on a screen is itself part of the communication dialog. User testing must be a sustained and crucial part of interface development to be sure that, collectively, the information roll-out of products from an informatics program has the intended effect in enabling effective policy. The information on the screen, though crucial, will constitute only one part of the total communication impact from a successful informatics program. Focus group testing and stakeholder interviews can be conducted to improve the strategic impact of press releases and printed reports. Depending on the complexity of the informatics program, ongoing user training might need to be offered to ensure that the data from the program are used accurately and are consistent with programmatic goals.

Conclusion

The SEER registry data presented at the beginning of this chapter paint a picture of unequal distribution of health benefits from the scientific advances made in preventing, detecting, and treating cancer (Grann et al., 2006; Jemal et al., 2004; Lathan, Neville, & Earle, 2006; Singh & Miller, 2003). The population pathways for addressing this inequality are undoubtedly complex, reflecting the insidious pervasiveness of poverty, illiteracy, and disenfranchisement (Demasio, 2003). Nevertheless, the population data add specificity to the problem. Just as bioimaging techniques and biomarkers give oncologists the tools they need to make physiological progress against a once unassailable disease, the SEER public health data are giving epidemiologists and policy makers the tools they need to accelerate the benefits of scientific knowledge equitably throughout the population. Already the program has given rise to policy changes that have saved countless lives nationally by providing for improved access to screening, public communication campaigns, and community outreach (Adams, Breen, & Joski, 2007; Tangka et al., 2006).

This chapter describes some of the contributions that pubic health informatics can make to the seemingly intractable problem of overcoming health disparities. It also describes an era of informatics research in which many of the driving questions have less to do with initiating new data collection programs, and more to do with making better use of the disconnected data systems that already exist. The goal is to move beyond the sense of "data smog" (Shenk, 1997) that is currently paralyzing action in the public health arena, to enable a clear path for evidence-based policy and intervention. Quite simply, it is time to accelerate progress in "connecting the dots" within existing public health data systems; lives are depending on it.

References

Abbas, A. (2004). *Grid computing: A practical guide to technology and applications.* Bingham, MA: Charles River Media, Inc.

Abrams, D. B. (1999). Transdisciplinary paradigms for tobacco prevention research. *Nicotine & Tobacco Research, 1*(Suppl. 1), S15–S23.

Abrams, D. B. (2006). Applying transdisciplinary research strategies to understanding and eliminating health disparities. *Health Education & Behavior, 33*, 515–531.

Adams, E. K., Breen, N., & Joski, P. J. (2007). Impact of the national breast and cervical cancer early detection program on mammography and Pap test utilization among White, Hispanic, and African American women: 1996–2000. *Cancer, 109*, 348–358.

Agresti, W. W. (2003). Discovery informatics. *Communications of the ACM, 46*, 25–28.

Atkins, D. E. (2003). *Revolutionizing science and engineering through cyberinfrastructure: Report of the national science foundation.* Blue ribbon advisory panel on cyberinfrastructure. Arlington, VA: National Science Foundation.

Benderson, B., & Schneiderman, B. (2003). *The craft of information visualization: Readings and reflections.* Boston: Morgan Kaufmann.

Boslaugh, S. E., Kreuter, M. W., Nicholson, R. A., & Naleid, K. (2005). Comparing demographic, health status and psychosocial strategies of audience segmentation to promote physical activity. *Health Education Research, 20*, 430–438.

Brailer, D. (2005). Action through collaboration: A conversation with David Brailer. Interview by Robert Cunningham. *Health Affairs (Project Hope), 24*, 1150–1157.

Broome, C. V., & Loonsk, J. (2004). Public health information network – Improving early detection by using a standards-based approach to connecting public health and clinical medicine. *MMWR. Morbidity and Mortality Weekly Report, 53*(Suppl.), 199–202.

Buetow, K. H. (2005). Cyberinfrastructure: Empowering a "third way" in biomedical research. *Science, 308*, 821–824.

Burrage, K., Hood, L., & Ragan, M. A. (2006). Advanced computing for systems biology. *Briefings in Bioinformatics, 7*, 390–398.

Cancer facts and figures 2006. (2006a). Washington, DC: American Cancer Society.

Cassa, C. A., Grannis, S. J., Overhage, J. M., & Mandl, K. D. (2006). A context-sensitive approach to anonymizing spatial surveillance data: Impact on outbreak detection. *Journal of the American Medical Informatics Association, 13*, 160–165.

Chueh, H. C., & Barnett, G. O. (1994). Client–server, distributed database strategies in a healthcare record system for a homeless population. *Journal of the American Medical Informatics Association, 1*, 186–198.

Chute, C. G., Cohn, S. P., & Campbell, J. R. (1998). A framework for comprehensive health terminology systems in the United States: Development guidelines, criteria for selection, and public policy implications. ANSI Healthcare Informatics Standards Board Vocabulary Working Group and the Computer-Based Patient Records Institute Working Group on Codes and Structures. *Journal of the American Medical Informatics Association, 5*, 503–510.

Clancy, C. M., & Scully, T. (2003). A call to excellence. *Health Affairs (Project Hope), 22*, 113–115.

Committee on the review and assessment of the NIH's Strategic Research Plan and Budget to Reduce and Ultimately Eliminate Health Disparities. (2007). *Examining the health disparities research plan of the National Institutes of Health: Unfinished business.* Washington, DC: The National Academy Press.

Culliton, B. J. (2006). Extracting knowledge from science: A conversation with Elias Zerhouni. *Health Affairs (Project Hope), 25*(3), w94–w103.

Demasio, K. A. (2003). The complexity of finding solutions to reducing racial/ethnic disparities in health care outcomes. Commentary on "A community approach to addressing excess breast and cervical cancer mortality among women of African descent in Boston". *Public Health Reports, 118*, 348.

Edwards, B. K., Brown, M. L., Wingo, P. A., Howe, H. L., Ward, E., Ries, L. A., et al. (2005). Annual report to the nation on the status of cancer, 1975–2002, featuring population-based trends in cancer treatment. *Journal of the National Cancer Institute, 97*, 1407–1427.

Ellisman, M., Brady, M., Hart, D., Lin, F.-P., Muller, M., & Smarr, L. (2004). The emerging role of biogrids. *Communications of the ACM, 47*, 53–56.

Freidman, T. L. (2006). *The world is flat a brief history of the twenty-first century*. New York: Farrar, Strauss and Giroux.

Freimuth, V. S. (1993). Narrowing the cancer knowledge gap between whites and African Americans. *Journal of the National Cancer Institute. Monographs, 14*, 81–91.

Fulcher, C. L., & Kaukinen, C. E. (2004). Visualizing the infrastructure of US healthcare using Internet GIS: A community health informatics approach for reducing health disparities. MEDINFO, *11*, 1197–1201.

Gibbons, M. C. (2005). A historical overview of health disparities and the potential of eHealth solutions. *Journal of Medical Internet Research, 7*, e50.

Gibbons, M. C. (2006). Health inequalities and emerging themes in compunetics. *Studies in Health Technology and Informatics, 121*, 62–69.

Grann, V., Troxel, A. B., Zojwalla, N., Hershman, D., Glied, S. A., & Jacobson, J. S. (2006). Regional and racial disparities in breast cancer-specific mortality. *Social Science & Medicine, 62*, 337–347.

Hanchette, C. L. (2003). Geographic information systems. In P. W. O'Carrol, W. A. Yasnoff, M. E. Ward, L. H. Ripp, & E. L. Martin (Eds.), *Public health informatics and information systems* (pp. 431–466). New York: Springer.

Hankey, B. F., Ries, L. A., & Edwards, B. K. (1999). The surveillance, epidemiology, and end results program: A national resource. *Cancer Epidemiology, Biomarkers & Prevention, 8*, 1117–1121.

Hesse, B. W. (2005). Harnessing the power of an intelligent health environment in cancer control. *Studies in Health Technology Informatics, 118*, 159–176.

Hesse, B. W., & Schneiderman, B. (in press). eHealth research from the user's perspective. *American Journal of Preventive Medicine*.

Hiatt, R. A., & Rimer, B. K. (1999). A new strategy for cancer control research. *Cancer Epidemiology, Biomarkers & Prevention, 8*, 957–964.

Howe, H. L., Edwards, B. K., Young, J. L., Shen, T., West, D. W., Hutton, M., et al. (2003). A vision for cancer incidence surveillance in the United States. *Cancer Causes & Control, 14*, 663–672.

IOM Committee on Quality of Healthcare in America. (2001). *Crossing the quality chasm: A new health system for the 21st century*. Washington, DC: The National Academy Press.

James, B. (2005). E-health: Steps on the road to interoperability. *Health Affairs (Project Hope)*, Suppl. Web Exclusives, W5.

Jemal, A., Clegg, L. X., Ward, E., Ries, L. A., Wu, X., Jamison, P. M., et al. (2004). Annual report to the nation on the status of cancer, 1975–2001, with a special feature regarding survival. *Cancer, 101*, 3–27.

Jernigan, D. B., Davies, J., & Sim, A. (2003). Data standards in public health informatics. In P. W. O'Carrol, W. A. Yasnoff, M. E. Ward, L. H. Ripp, & E. L. Martin (Eds.), *Public health informatics and information systems* (pp. 213–238). New York: Springer.

Kass-Hout, T. A., Gray, S. K., Massoudi, B. L., Immanuel, G. Y., Dollacker, M., & Cothren, R. (2007). NHIN, RHIOs, and public health. *Journal of Public Health Management and Practice, 13*, 31–34.

Koo, D., O'Carroll, P., & LaVenture, M. (2001). Public health 101 for informaticians. *Journal of the American Medical Informatics Association, 8*, 585–597.

Lathan, C. S., Neville, B. A., & Earle, C. C. (2006). The effect of race on invasive staging and surgery in non-small-cell lung cancer. *Journal of Clinical Oncology, 24*, 413–418.

Litt, J. S., Tran, N. L., & Burke, T. A. (2002). Examining urban brownfields through the public health "macroscope". *Environmental Health Perspectives, 110*(Suppl. 2), 183–193.

Lumpkin, J. R. (2003). History and significance of information systems in public health. In P. W. O'Carrol, W. A. Yasnoff, M. E. Ward, L. H. Ripp, & E. L. Martin (Eds.), *Public health informatics and information systems* (pp. 16–38). New York: Springer.

Mandl, K. D., & Lee, T. H. (2002). Integrating medical informatics and health services research: The need for dual training at the clinical health systems and policy levels. *Journal of the American Medical Informatics Association, 9*, 127–132.

National Center for Health Statistics. (2001). *Information for health: A strategy for building the National Health Information Infrastructure.* Washington, DC: DHHS.

National Committee in Vital and Health Statistics. (2005). *Eliminating health disparities: Strengthening data on race, ethnicity, and primary language in the United States.* Washington, DC: DHHS.

OBSSR, N. N. N. (2006). *Stress and coping: Matrices for cross-center collaborations.* Washington, DC: DHHS.

O'Carroll, P. W. (2003). Introduction to public health informatics. In P. W. O'Carrol (Ed.), *Public health informatics and information systems* (pp. 3–15). New York: Springer.

Pestell, R. (2006). Remembering team science is for the patients. *Cancer Biology & Therapy, 5*, 449–452.

Safran, C. (2003). The collaborative edge: Patient empowerment for vulnerable populations. *International Journal of Medical Informatics, 69*, 185–190.

Safran, C., Bloomrosen, M., Hammond, W. E., Labkoff, S., Markel-Fox, S., Tang, P. C., et al. (2007). Toward a national framework for the secondary use of health data: An American Medical Informatics Association White Paper. *Journal of the American Medical Informatics Association, 14*, 1–9.

Sellers, T. A., Caporaso, N., Lapidus, S., Petersen, G. M., & Trent, J. (2006). Opportunities and barriers in the age of team science: Strategies for success. *Cancer Causes & Control, 17*, 229–237.

Shenk, D. (1997). *Data smog: Surviving the information glut* (1st ed.). San Fransisco: Harper Edge.

Shortliffe, E. H., & Sondik, E. J. (2006). The public health informatics infrastructure: Anticipating its role in cancer. *Cancer Causes & Control, 17*, 861–869.

Silent Victories: The history and practice of public health in twentieth-century America. (2006b). New York: Oxford University Press.

Singh, G., & Miller, B. (2003). *Area socioeconomic variations in US cancer incidence, mortality, stage, treatment and survival, 1975–1999 (Rep. No. NIH 03–5417).* Bethesda, MD: National Cancer Institute.

Snee, N. L., & McCormick, K. A. (2004). The case for integrating public health informatics networks. *IEEE Engineering in Medicine and Biology Magazine, 23*, 81–88.

Strunk, R. C., Ford, J. G., & Taggart, V. (2002). Reducing disparities in asthma care: Priorities for research – National Heart, Lung, and Blood Institute workshop report. *The Journal of Allergy and Clinical Immunology, 109*, 229–237.

Tangka, F. K., Dalaker, J., Chattopadhyay, S. K., Gardner, J. G., Royalty, J., Hall, I. J., et al. (2006). Meeting the mammography screening needs of underserved women: The performance of the National Breast and Cervical Cancer Early Detection Program in 2002–2003 (United States). *Cancer Causes & Control, 17*, 1145–1154.

Viswanath, K., Breen, N., Meissner, H., Moser, R. P., Hesse, B., Steele, W. R., et al. (2006). Cancer knowledge and disparities in the information age. *Journal of Health Communication, 11*(Suppl. 1), 1–17.

Weir, H. K., Thun, M. J., Hankey, B. F., Ries, L. A., Howe, H. L., Wingo, P. A., et al. (2003). Annual report to the nation on the status of cancer, 1975–2000, featuring the uses of surveillance data for cancer prevention and control. *Journal of the National Cancer Institute, 95*, 1276–1299.

Wingo, P. A., Howe, H. L., Thun, M. J., Ballard-Barbash, R., Ward, E., Brown, M. L., et al. (2005). A national framework for cancer surveillance in the United States. *Cancer Causes & Control, 16*, 151–170.

Yasnoff, W. A., & Miller, P. L. (2003). Discision support and expert systems. In P. W. O'Carrol, W. A. Yasnoff, M. E. Ward, L. H. Ripp, & E. L. Martin (Eds.), *Public health informatics and information systems* (pp. 16–38). New York: Springer.

Zerhouni, E. A. (2005, March 9). *Testimony before the house appropriations subcommittee on labor/HHS & education.* Bethesda, MD: National Institutes of Health.

Section IV

12
Beyond Traditional Paradigms in Disparities Research

M. Chris Gibbons, Malcolm Brock, Anthony J Alberg, Thomas Glass, Thomas A LaVeist, Stephen Baylin, David Levine, and C. Earl Fox

Introduction

Recently several researchers have hypothesized pathways that attempt to explain how the sociobehavioral environment is related to health and health disparities (Acheson, 1998; Adler & Ostrove, 1999; Baum, Garofalo, & Yali, 1999; Birch, 1999; Capitman, Bhalotra, Calderon-Rosado, & Gibbons, 2003; Fuhrer et al., 2002; Macintyre, 1997; Macintyre, Ellaway, & Cummins, 2002; Williams, 1999). Historically these conceptual frameworks have formed a solid foundation upon which science has been built. Upon review of these frameworks, it is possible to make at least three general observations. The first is the lack of depth to which they integrate our present understanding of the biology of disease, particularly at the cellular and molecular levels. With the exception of those pathways based on stress (neuroimmunological) mechanisms, the published frameworks in the behavioral sciences and epidemiological literature largely lack clearly stated, causal biologic connections to observed health outcomes (Acheson; Adler & Ostrove; Evans & Stoddart, 1990; LaLonde, 1981; Macintyre; Williams). On the other hand, the biologically oriented formulations poorly account for socioenvironmental and behavioral effect modifiers that may affect the pathogenesis of disease and the development of health disparities (Burger & Gimelfarb, 1999; Meyer & Breitner, 1998; Phillips & Belknap, 2002; Sharma, 1998).

Secondly, the terminology used to characterize the effects of causal agents are poorly standardized with substantial blurring of concepts derived from toxicology, biostatistics, epidemiology, sociology (Baron & Kenny, 1986), and the clinical/bench sciences (Minamoto, Mai, & Ronai, 1999; Stucker et al., 2002). Across these fields, the terms cause, mediator, moderator, regulator, effector, interaction and mechanism of action have vastly different meanings, which may not be readily apparent to all investigators. For example epidemiologists and statisticians tend to use the terms mediators and moderators to describe distinct aspects of an observed association between two independent variables, largely without reference to the

Reprinted with permission from the Journal of Urban Health, 84(2), March, 2007, Springer.

underlying biophysiologic processes. On the other hand, toxicologists and clinical/bench scientists tend to use the terms mediators, moderators, and regulators almost synonymously as descriptors of factors, substances, or agents that alter some characteristic of a known or unknown biophysiologic mechanism. They also tend to reserve the term "cause" or "causal pathway" to describe an agent or series of biophysiologic events that must occur to result in a given outcome.

Finally, scientists and investigators trained in the clinical and bench sciences generally consider discreet, quantitative exposures (viral, bacterial, toxicological, psychological, etc.) as the etiologic agents of disease. Historically these exposures have been studied in isolation from the broader sociobehavioral contexts in which they exist. On the other hand social scientists often consider more qualitative social factors like poverty, socioeconomic status, and racial segregation as the key determinants of health (Berkman & Kawachi, 2000; LaVeist, 2002). They often assert that other more quantitative exposures are factors which alter the nature of the association between the social factor and a given health outcome (Amick, Levine, Tarlov, & Walsh, 1995). When social scientists are describing causal factors, they draw a distinction between proximal social factors which they define as the settings in which people live (family, work, school, and neighborhood) and distal social factors, which they define as, the pervasive forces in society (culture, socioeconomic status, and race relations) (Amick et al.).

The unique perspectives of each scientific discipline have both strengths and weaknesses. However, as transdisciplinary investigation is increasingly undertaken, the resultant confusion in scientific discourse may hinder scientific inquiry and the advance of knowledge.

Given this level of complexity, a sociobiologic organizing model or framework could enhance the nascent link between sociobehavioral investigation and biophysiologic or biomolecular mechanisms. Attempts to organize and understand complex biologic systems have been attempted in the past. Some researchers have looked to Chaos theory and Complexity theory as constructs to facilitating understanding about health and its relationship to diverse processes and outcomes such as cardiac arrhythmias (Garfinkel, Spano, Ditto, & Weiss, 1992; Weiss, Garfinkel, Spano, & Ditto, 1994) and even urban epidemics (Olsen & Schaffer, 1990; Tidd, Olsen, & Schaffer, 1993). While this approach may have merit, it appears to be beyond the practical usefulness of many clinicians and scientists.

The inherent difficulty of developing a useful transdisciplinary model is demonstrated by the fact that any model detailing all possible biologic pathways through which all possible social and behavioral factors impact all possible health outcomes would be exceedingly complex. Alternatively, an overly simplistic model would likewise be of little value (Berkman & Kawachi, 2000). The goal of this paper is to articulate a framework through which multilevel, transdisciplinary, work might be collectively organized.

In this paper, an exhaustive analysis or critique of the science is not attempted. Rather, at each step of our model we will provide illustrative examples that suggest how information from disparate fields might be integrated within a single biologically plausible, mechanistically driven, multilevel framework.

The SBIM

In brief, the SBIM suggests that individuals are constantly being exposed to many health-impacting environmental inputs. These inputs are often modified to increase or attenuate their effects via other "indirect" environmental inputs. Both direct and indirect inputs are in turn, acted upon by metabolic, digestive, and or detoxification systems often producing measurable biologic products (biomarkers). If inputs or metabolic products overwhelm bodily defense or regulatory mechanisms, disease will occur. Because inputs, biologic processes, and outcomes exist on several levels, the model is conceived as operating on the cellular, individual, and population levels, temporally proceeding from input (exposure) to outcome (Fig. 12.1).

As applied to our model, the term "environmental" is used in a broad sense. It includes factors such as toxicological agents, microbial pathogens as well as socio-cultural and geopolitical influences. Because these exposures are extremely varied and emanate from many very different types of sources, we refer to them collectively as inputs. Specifically we define direct inputs as those exposures that directly alter normal host DNA (Directly Causal). In contrast to direct inputs, many exposures impact host physiology only indirectly, albeit at times profoundly. Examples of these types of indirectly acting exposures would include culture and socioeconomic status. We define these indirectly acting factors as indirect environmental inputs.

Population level direct inputs would include certain carcinogenic emissions from urban factories or diesel exhaust fumes among inner city residents and workers. Individual level direct inputs would include such things as alcohol- and food-based carcinogen exposures. Finally cellular direct inputs would include tumor suppressor genes, which confer increased susceptibility of cancer on those who possess the genes.

As with direct inputs, indirect inputs exist on the cellular, individual, and population levels (Amick et al., 1995; Berkman & Kawachi, 2000; Braunwald et al., 2001; Christenson & Azzazy, 1998; Evans, Barer, & Marmor, 1994; Minamoto et al., 1999; Pargament, Maton, & Hess, 1992; Wadsworth, 1997). For example, tobacco regulatory policies may function as population-level indirect inputs that impact cigarette carcinogen exposure. Thus, people who work in smoke-free environments would potentially be exposed to less work-related tobacco carcinogens than those working in smoke-filled workplaces. Individual level indirect inputs include gender, age, host immune status, health literacy, and family or social networks. Social networks, for example, impact health outcomes because individuals with larger, more robust social networks tend to engage in health-promoting behaviors and to avoid health-damaging behaviors (Cattell, 2001). Finally, other indirect inputs such as genetic polymorphisms of tumor associated genes, operate at the cellular or molecular level, impacting gene function or expression (Friedman & Lawrence, 2002; Goldman & Shields, 2003; Kelada et al., 2000; Kramer et al., 2001; Minamoto et al., 1999; Mucci, Wedren, Tamimi, Trichopoulos, & Adami, 2001; Slattery et al., 2002; Ulrich et al., 1999; Wilson, Jones, Coussens, & Hanna, 2002) (see lung cancer discussion below).

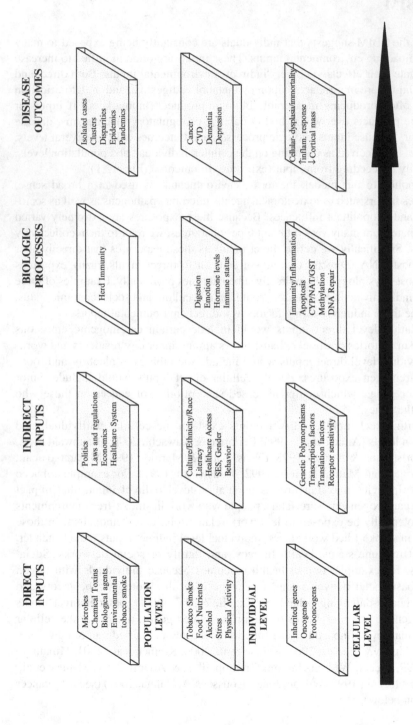

Fig. 12.1. This graphic depicts the SBIM. It shows the general temporal relationship between exposures (inputs), factors which can alter these exposures (mediators), biophysiologic mechanisms impacted by these exposures, and potential observed outcomes on the population, individual, and cellular levels

The specific group of direct and indirect inputs to which an individual is exposed may be highly variable between individuals or populations. Ultimately it is determined by the sociocultural milieu or surroundings in which the individual lives, works, and socializes.

After being altered by indirect inputs, all inputs (direct and indirect) are acted upon by one or more degradory, detoxification, immune or metabolic systems or biologic processes within the body. These systems include, but are not limited to, the N-acetyltransferase enzymes, the Phase I cytochrome p450 system, and the Phase II glutathione-S-transferase system (Mucci et al., 2001). Although there are potentially many such systems operating in the body, the absolute number is finite. Integratively understanding health then, requires that the combined effects of all inputs (direct and indirect) be understood in the context of their impact on biologic processes.

During these processes, a myriad of excretory, secretory, respiratory, hormonal, and other metabolic substances are produced. Many of these substances are potential biomarkers. Biomarkers have become central to clinical medicine, pathology, and molecular epidemiology. Some biomarkers have utility in the diagnosis, treatment, and follow-up of disease. The utility of many others is under active investigation (Andreasen & Blennow, 2002; Christenson & Azzazy, 1998; De Servi, La Porta, Bontempelli, & Comolli, 2002; Kharitonov & Barnes, 2001; Meyer & Ginsburg, 2002; Montuschi et al., 2000; Pitot, 2002b).

Finally, the SBIM posits that disease will only occur if the magnitude of impact produced by inputs and metabolic processes is sufficient to overwhelm bodily reparative, restorative, or compensatory mechanisms, causing the accumulation of genotypic, phenotypic, or psychologic abnormalities which ultimately result in a disease state or health deficit. The challenge then for science is to use this model first to help organize and define the inputs, biologic processes, and outcomes that exist on each of the three suggested levels of exposure. The second challenge is to define how each of these factors relates to each other, again within the framework of a causal schema, to produce the outcome of interest. In other words elucidate the relationships between inputs, processes, and outcomes to produce the individual level outcome (disease) or population level outcome (disparity) of interest.

Lung Cancer and the SBIM

The SBIM framework suggests that the development of lung cancer is preceded by one or more carcinogenic direct inputs (exposures). Environmental, behavioral, and occupational exposures to well-known pulmonary carcinogens including tobacco, asbestos, radon, polycyclic aromatic hydrocarbons (PAHs), and heterocyclic amines are well documented (Alberg & Samet, 2003; Franceschi & Bidoli, 1999; Pitot, 2002b) (Fig. 12.2).

Next, indirect inputs modify these exposures. Potential indirect inputs of pulmonary carcinogens are many and as indicated by the model, operate on the cellular, individual, and population levels. Population level indirect inputs could include

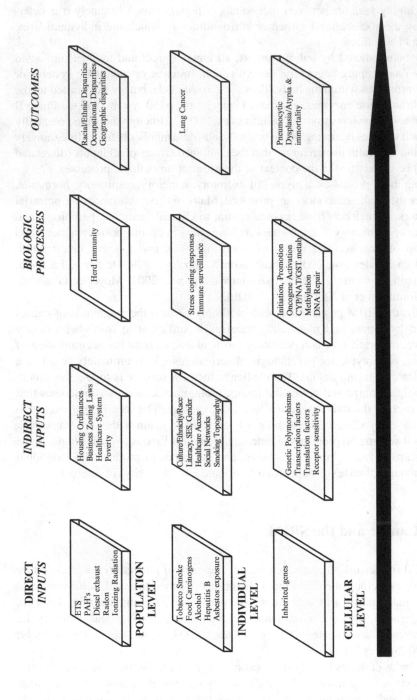

Fig. 12.2. This graphic employs the SBIM to outline a mechanistically driven framework for understanding socioenvironmentally associated lung cancer development on the cellular, individual, and population levels

certain geographic factors such as physical proximity of housing to a source of ambient air particulate toxicants. Individuals living in housing units located close to a factory spewing carcinogenic emissions from its smoke stack might be expected to experience higher carcinogenic exposure levels over time as compared to ambient air exposures in individuals who live farther away from these sites. In fact, location of urban residence has been associated with increased personal exposure and an increased lifetime risk of cancer (Kinney, Chillrud, Ramstrom, Ross, & Stansfeld, 2002; Morello-Frosch, Pastor, Porras, & Sadd, 2002). In addition, carcinogenic exposures from other sources like diesel exhaust fumes may be significantly higher in urban communities than exposures to these same carcinogens in rural environments. Scientific evidence does indeed document that the carcinogenic activity of some PAHs may be related to exposures not only from cigarettes, but also from other environmental sources (Hecht, 1999). Coke oven plant workers, commercial printers, truckers (diesel exhaust), and workers from rubber, asphalt, coal, and aluminum plants are all at increased risk of exposure to PAHs (Benowitz, 1997; Fielding, Husten, & Eriksen, 1998; Morello-Frosch et al., 2002). Occupational scientists have shown that increased work-related PAH exposure is associated with an increased risk of morbidity (Kyle, Woodruff, Buffler, & Davis, 2002), DNA damage (Sorenson et al., 2003), abnormal methylation of tumor-associated genes (Belinsky et al., 2002), and increased risk of lung cancer (Pope et al., 2002; Zmirou, Masclet, Boudet, Dor, & Dechenaux, 2000). Thus both proximity of urban residence to a carcinogenic source and ambient air toxicant concentrations likely influence cumulative individual and population PAH exposure.

As one continues to think about potential lung cancer indirect inputs, the role of diet as an important factor must be considered. While diet has often been considered an important carcinogenic exposure, the SBIM encourages a more explicit understanding of diet, dietary constituent, and their level of exposure. As such it may be that specific dietary nutrients or dietary carcinogens would be considered inputs, while other sociocultural and regulatory factors that influence or influence dietary choices of individuals would be considered indirect inputs. As such "diet" may be considered a culturally influenced (and as such population level) indirect input while the actual dietary constituents consumed may be seen as an individual level direct or indirect input or depending on the specific constituent in question. For example, cruciferous vegetables of the *Brassica* family (broccoli, cauliflower, etc.) have been linked to their ability to effect the activity of CYP and GST enzymatic systems thereby inhibiting phase I bioactivation of carcinogens and inducing phase II carcinogenic detoxification (Weisburger & Chung, 2002; Yang, Chhabra, Hong, & Smith, 2001; Zhao et al., 2001). Thus broccoli in the diet would be an individual level indirect input, while the availability of broccoli at local grocery stores, the price of broccoli in those stores, or whether or not individuals would choose to eat broccoli would on the other hand represent societal (neighborhood), SES (market forces dictating prices), cultural (certain cultures tend not to eat certain things) factors which in the SBIM framework would all represent population level indirect inputs.

Local or national regulatory policy may also influence lung carcinogenesis at the population level by either indirectly influencing dietary food choices or by influencing carcinogenic exposures among populations. For example, consider that grocery store location, cost of foodstuffs, and quality of supermarkets have all been linked to dietary choices and nutrient availability (Morland, Wing, & Diez, 2002). In the case of liquor establishments, store location and number of stores in a given community have been shown to be associated with amount of alcohol ingested per capita in the local community and associated with dietary nutrient intake by local community residents (LaVeist & Wallace, 2000). Regulatory policies then, such as business zoning and liquor licensing laws, may have the unintentional and unrecognized consequences of influencing cancer risk by impacting personal ambient air carcinogenic exposures via regulating the proximity and density of living establishments to urban and occupational particulate carcinogen sources and by influencing dietary nutrient availability of residents living in a given community.

Finally, in terms of indirect inputs, the carcinogenic potential of the PAHs may be impacted by the presence or absence of a given genetic polymorphism operating on the cellular level (Alexandrov et al., 2002; Haugen et al., 2000; Itoga et al., 2002; Kamataki, Nunoya, Sakai, Kushida, & Fujita, 1999; Lewis, Cherry, Niven, Barber, & Povey, 2002; Miller et al., 2002; Shields, 1999; Song, Tan, Xing, & Lin, 2001; Stucker et al., 2002; Sunaga et al., 2002). Researchers then could seek to elucidate the relationships between these multilevel phenomenon which all operate along the lung cancer causal chain in individuals, to produce lung cancer or not and also among populations to produce a given lung cancer disparity.

It is true that completely characterizing the independent and joint effects of all potential direct and indirect inputs in complex mixtures such as ambient air, tobacco smoke, and diet, or completely quantifying the effects of all important genes and polymorphisms impacting biologic all requisite biologic processes is a formidable task (Feron & Groten, 2002; Mauderly, 1993; Samet, 1995). However, it is clear that as many social and environmental sources as possible must be collectively considered, evaluated, and quantified in order to most accurately ascertain, cumulative individual and community level carcinogenic exposure or risk.

Continuing with our model, the physiologic disposition of carcinogenic inputs occurs next. Here, the biomolecular experimental literature is replete with relevant mechanisms and several excellent reviews summarize the expansive current knowledge of biochemical and molecular genetic events involved in the metabolism of tobacco carcinogens (Medelsohn, Howley, Isreal, & Liotta, 2001; Pitot, 2002a; Schuller, 2002; Terry, 1964; Zochbauer-Muller, Gazdar, & Minna, 2002). As such, these will not be detailed. In brief though, over time, prolonged tobacco-related carcinogenic exposure is associated with progressive accumulation of phenotypic and genotypic abnormalities, leading to tumor initiation, promotion, and progression (Medelsohn et al.; Pitot, 2002a; Schuller, 2002; Terry; Zochbauer-Muller et al.). Consequent to these processes, many metabolites and byproducts are produced, released, or otherwise given off. Recent advances in molecular biology and genetics have made it possible to identify many of these potential lung cancer biomarkers

(Hecht, 2002; Meyer & Ginsburg, 2002). The relative utility of these biomarkers in cancer prevention and prognostication is an active area of research.

Finally, according to the SBIM lung cancer will occur if the *combined effects of all important* carcinogenic direct and indirect inputs are sufficient to cause the accumulation of phenotypic and genotypic abnormalities, such that tumor initiation, promotion, and progression will occur in individuals (disease) or populations (disparity). Thus as can be seen from the preceding example a single organizing framework such as the SBIM is needed to help organize the myriad of factors involved in lung cancer susceptibility, occurrence among individuals, or to comprehensively explain differential outcomes between populations.

Health Disparities, Lung Cancer, and the SBIM

Given that the human genome has proven to be highly conserved, genotypic variation alone cannot adequately explain the existence of health disparities and socioenvironmental factors are now believed to be important in their development. In general, the SBIM model suggests that health disparities (a population level outcome) occur when direct input-indirect input profiles (the sum total of the effects of all inputs) are sufficient to produce disease (lung cancer) in a higher than expected number of individuals in a given population. With regards to lung cancer specifically, the interplay of environmental factors, geography, smoking, and biology suggested by the SBIM may underlie findings such as those of Pastorino et al. who studied the relationship between occupational carcinogen exposure and cigarette smoking in lung cancer. His work found that in a general industrial worker population, occupational exposure to pulmonary carcinogens causes lung cancer in a cooperative and multiplicative fashion with increasing levels of cigarette smoking (Pastorino et al., 1984). Archer, Wagoner, and Lundin (1973) reported similar findings among uranium miners who smoked. These studies demonstrated that occupational exposures conferred an increased risk of lung cancer in smokers and nonsmokers. This elevated risk, however, was further increased, exponentially with increasing levels of cigarette smoking. Thinking about these observations within the context of the SBIM, it would suggest a more explicit characterization of known inputs (direct and indirect) and biologic processes, their level of influence and path (do these inputs exert effects only on one level of influence or multiple levels, what is the differential strength of influence on the various levels) of influence is needed to fully understand these observations.

Racial and ethnic disparities in lung cancer offer another illustrative case in point. According to the recent SEER data, African-American men have significantly elevated lung cancer incidence and mortality rates as compared to white males. African-American females on the other hand have only a slightly elevated lung cancer incidence and essentially the same lung cancer mortality rate as compared to white women (*Cancer facts and figures 2003*, 2003a) (Table 12.1).

Table 12.1. Recent SEER data depicting current racial and ethnic lung cancer disparities between African-Americans and Whites in lung cancer incidence and mortality

US lung cancer incidence and mortality rates, 1992–1999

	White	African-American
Lung cancer incidence		
Males	82.9	124.1
Females	51.1	53.2
Total	64.3	82.6
Lung cancer mortality		
Males	81.7	113.0
Females	41.1	39.6
Total	57.9	68.9

At first, no readily apparent, biologically plausible explanation for these findings is evident. The SBIM may suggest some scientific lines of inquiry or indicate some potential pathways. Indeed it is true that many causal pathways likely contribute to the observed population epidemiology. Additionally as stated above, accurate and precise risk characterization can only be accomplished after accounting for all environmental sources of pulmonary carcinogens and major mediators. Finally, causal pathways must work through biological mechanisms.

The SBIM suggests that at a minimum, precise lung cancer risk characterization must include an assessment of tobacco smoking patterns, geographic factors, occupational exposures, and major potential mediators. With regard to smoking habits, 2001 National Health Interview Survey data reveal that among working age individuals, overall smoking rates do not significantly differ between non-Hispanic African-Americans and non-Hispanic Whites. The data also indicate that only relatively small gender differences in smoking prevalence exist (Male = 2.7, 95% CI 23.9–254.6, Female = 20.8, 95% CI 20.1–21.5, White = 24.5% CI 23.8–25.2, African-American = 22.2% CI 22.1–23.3) (*Early release of selected estimates based on data from the 2001 National Health Interview Survey*, 2003b). Epidemiologic data evaluating smoking trends in the US over the last three decades revealed that the prevalence of current smoking has consistently been highest among Blacks, in particular, black males, with generally lower rates for females (Garfinkel, 1997; Zang & Wynder, 1998). Men generally smoked more cigarettes per day than females, but overall Whites smoke more cigarettes than Blacks (Garfinkel; Zang & Wynder). Recent increases in smoking by African-American females, however, have led to cigarette consumption rates on par with African-American men. Despite the higher number of cigarettes smoked by Caucasians, most African-Americans smoke the brands with higher tar yields per cigarette (Zang & Wynder). Finally, in the 1960s and 1970s the age at smoking initiation for women was approximately 4 years later than men. By the 1990s this difference had been reduced to 2 years (Zang & Wynder). Thus although cigarette smoking is associated with the majority of lung cancer cases today, epidemiologic evaluation of historic smoking patterns in the US do not easily help to explain racial differences in lung cancer incidence and mortality. Potential other factors including occupation and place of residence may be important in the genesis of observed lung cancer disparities.

Racial and ethnic minority workers are generally overrepresented in blue collar and service jobs while underrepresented in professional careers (Murray, 2003). In many of these jobs, minority workers are differentially exposed to occupational carcinogens, resulting in disproportionate disease (Luepker et al., 1994). Also significant proportions of racial and ethnic minority workers live in central cities, in close geographic proximity to industrial plants or factories. Finally males comprise the majority of workers who work in exposure-prone industries (miners, steel workers, and chemical industry workers). Individually, these findings do not suggest a unified causal pathway. However, by employing the SBIM to collectively understand how these contributing factors collectively may impact tumor biology, biologically plausible clues begin to emerge.

One possible pathway that is suggested by the SBIM is that differential exposures related to urban residence and occupation across racial and ethnic groups may act cooperatively to influence the genesis of lung cancer disparities. For example, at baseline, men smoke more than women and Blacks smoke higher tar-yielding cigarettes as compared to Whites. In addition this smoking related risk elevation in African-Americans might be further heightened via ambient air carcinogenic exposures among African-Americans who live in the urban inner city. This could further elevate the risk of lung cancer in African-Americans above that of White Americans who are less likely to live in neighborhoods with elevated baseline ambient air carcinogen levels or smoke high tar cigarettes. Among males, African-American incidence and mortality rates may be still further increased through occupational carcinogenic exposures, which biologically act synergistically with smoking patterns and geographic exposures. Women, both African-American and Caucasian American who comprise a substantially smaller proportion of the workers in exposure-prone industries, would not have this additional exposure and thus may not be expected to have lung cancer incidence and mortality rates on par with African-American males. Finally, indirect inputs including insurance status, healthcare access, dietary factors, genetic polymorphisms, or regulatory policy may attenuate or potentiate this pathway as outlined in previous sections.

Discussion

Increasingly, scientific evidence suggests that disease causation in general and health disparities in particular, result from complex interactions of many factors which simultaneously and often cooperatively act across more than one level of influence over time. An integrated understanding of disease or disparities causation would likely facilitate research and breakthroughs in treatments and interventions. Achieving such a goal is in the current state of scientific inquiry is itself a difficult task, with several factors mitigating against such an accomplishment.

We first outline a multilevel, transdisciplinary organizing model and define the terminology used in reference to this model. Then using lung cancer as a case in point, we attempt to illustrate that this model provides a population-oriented, biologically grounded framework for understanding cancer etiology and pathogenesis. We also use the model to provide a mechanistic framework for understanding lung cancer disparities.

This model facilitates cross-disciplinary investigation and communication by providing a common conceptual model and terminology while articulating a biologically driven construct employing both sociobehavioral and biologic variables that influence disease pathogenesis. We acknowledge that some investigators will favor further subdivisions at each of the proposed levels of organization presented in this model. For example social scientists may prefer that the population level be subdivided into family, neighborhood, and community levels. On the other hand clinical scientists may want the individual level to be further subdivided into an "organ" level, while molecular scientists may seek a submolecular level to be added to the model. While each of these modifications may make sense to a given investigator, they also may have no meaning to an investigator who works largely on a different level. For example, social scientists may not see a reason or value of further subdividing the individual or cellular levels of the model while molecular scientists may see no need for multiple subdivisions at the population level. Indeed further subdivisions of the basic model may increase confusion *across* disciplines. As such, this model presents a basic three-level framework. Yet the authors vigorously encourage individual scientists and groups to further subdivide the model as deemed appropriate to facilitate their investigations. In this way it is hoped that this model may help science to move beyond only attempting to identify isolated "causes" of disease or isolated "causes" of health disparities (be they behavioral, biologic, or environmental), to also seeking to uncover *patterns* of behavior–biology interaction that positively or negatively affect individuals and populations. In so doing we may then improve our understanding of health and disease at the interface of biology, behavior, and the environment.

References

Acheson, D. (1998). *Independent inquiry into inequalities in health*. London: The Stationery Office.

Adler, N. E., & Ostrove, J. M. (1999). Socioeconomic status and health: What we know and what we don't. *Annals of the New York Academy of Sciences, 896*, 3–15.

Alberg, A. J., & Samet, J. M. (2003). Epidemiology of lung cancer. *Chest, 123*, 21S–49S.

Alexandrov, K., Cascorbi, I., Rojas, M., Bouvier, G., Kriek, E., & Bartsch, H. (2002). CYP1A1 and GSTM1 genotypes affect benzo[a]pyrene DNA adducts in smokers' lung: Comparison with aromatic/hydrophobic adduct formation. *Carcinogenesis, 23*, 1969–1977.

Amick, B. C., Levine, S., Tarlov, A. R., & Walsh, D. C. (1995). *Society and health*. New York: Oxford University Press.

Andreasen, N., & Blennow, K. (2002). Beta-amyloid (Abeta) protein in cerebrospinal fluid as a biomarker for Alzheimer's disease. *Peptides, 23*, 1205–1214.

Archer, V. E., Wagoner, J. K., & Lundin, F. E. (1973). Lung cancer among uranium miners in the United States. *Health Physics, 25,* 351–371.

Baron, R. M., & Kenny, D. A. (1986). The moderator–mediator variable distinction in social psychological research: Conceptual, strategic, and statistical considerations. *Journal of Personality and Social Psychology, 51,* 1173–1182.

Baum, A., Garofalo, J. P., & Yali, A. M. (1999). Socioeconomic status and chronic stress. Does stress account for SES effects on health? *Annals of the New York Academy of Sciences, 896,* 131–144.

Belinsky, S. A., Snow, S. S., Nikula, K. J., Finch, G. L., Tellez, C. S., & Palmisano, W. A. (2002). Aberrant CpG island methylation of the p16(INK4a) and estrogen receptor genes in rat lung tumors induced by particulate carcinogens. *Carcinogenesis, 23,* 335–339.

Benowitz, N. L. (1997). Smoking and occupational health. In J. Ladou (Ed.), *Occupational and environmental medicine* (2nd ed., pp. 713–722). Stamford, CT: Appleton and Lange.

Berkman, L. F., & Kawachi, I. (2000). *Social epidemiology.* New York: Oxford University Press.

Birch, S. (1999). The 39 steps: The mystery of health inequalities in the UK. *Health Economics, 8,* 301–308.

Braunwald, E., Jameson, J. L., Longo, D. L., Hauser, S. L., Kasper, D. L., & Fauci, A. S. (2001). *Harrisson's textbook of medicine* (15th ed.). New York: McGraw-Hill Publishers.

Burger, R., & Gimelfarb, A. (1999). Genetic variation maintained in multilocus models of additive quantitative traits under stabilizing selection. *Genetics, 152,* 807–820.

Cancer facts and figures 2003. (2003a). Washington, DC: American Cancer Society.

Capitman, J., Bhalotra, S. M., Calderon-Rosado, V., & Gibbons, M. C. (2003). *Cancer prevention and treatment demonstration for racial and ethnic minorities; Evidence report and evidence-based recommendations (Rep. No. 500-00-0031).* US Department of Health and Human Services.

Cattell, V. (2001). Poor people, poor places, and poor health: The mediating role of social networks and social capital. *Social Science & Medicine, 52,* 1501–1516.

Christenson, R. H., & Azzazy, H. M. (1998). Biochemical markers of the acute coronary syndromes. *Clinical Chemistry, 44,* 1855–1864.

De Servi, B., La Porta, C. A., Bontempelli, M., & Comolli, R. (2002). Decrease of TGF-beta1 plasma levels and increase of nitric oxide synthase activity in leukocytes as potential biomarkers of Alzheimer's disease.. Experimental Gerontology, *37,* 813–821.

Early release of selected estimates based on data from the 2001 National Health Interview Survey. (2003b). http://www.cdc.gov/nchs/about/major/nhis/released200207.htm#early [On-line].

Evans, R. G, Barer, M. L., & Marmor, T. R. (1994). *Why are some people healthy and others not? The determinants of population health.* New York: Aldine De Gruyter.

Evans, R. G., & Stoddart, G. L. (1990). Producing health, consuming health care. *Social Science & Medicine, 31,* 1347–1363.

Feron, V., & Groten, J. (2002). Toxicologic evaluation of chemical mixtures. *Food and Chemical Toxicology, 40,* 825–839.

Fielding, J. E., Husten, C. G., & Eriksen, M. P. (1998). Tobacco: Health effects and control. In R. B. Wallace (Ed.), *Public health and preventive medicine* (14th ed., pp. 817–846). Stamford, CT: Appleton and Lange.

Franceschi, S., & Bidoli, E. (1999). The epidemiology of lung cancer. *Annals of Oncology, 10*(Suppl. 5), S3–S6.

Friedman, E. M., & Lawrence, D. A. (2002). Environmental stress mediates changes in neuroimmunological interactions. *Toxicological Sciences, 67,* 4–10.

Fuhrer, R., Shipley, M. J., Chastang, J. F., Schmaus, A., Niedhammer, I., Stansfeld, S. A., et al. (2002). Socioeconomic position, health, and possible explanations: A tale of two cohorts. *American Journal of Public Health, 92,* 1290–1294.

Garfinkel, L. (1997). Trends in cigarette smoking in the United States. *Preventive Medicine, 26,* 447.

Garfinkel, A., Spano, M. L., Ditto, W. L., & Weiss, J. N. (1992). Controlling cardiac chaos. *Science, 257,* 1230–1235.

Goldman, R., & Shields, P. G. (2003). Food mutagens. *The Journal of Nutrition, 133*, 965S–973S.

Haugen, A., Ryberg, D., Mollerup, S., Zienolddiny, S., Skaug, V., & Svendsrud, D. H. (2000). Gene–environment interactions in human lung cancer. *Toxicology Letters, 112–113*, 233–237.

Hecht, S. S. (1999). Tobacco smoke carcinogens and lung cancer. *Journal of the National Cancer Institute, 91*, 1194–1210.

Hecht, S. S. (2002). Human urinary carcinogen metabolites: Biomarkers for investigating tobacco and cancer. *Carcinogenesis, 23*, 907–922.

Itoga, S., Nomura, F., Makino, Y., Tomonaga, T., Shimada, H., Ochiai, T., et al. (2002). Tandem repeat polymorphism of the CYP2E1 gene: An association study with esophageal cancer and lung cancer. *Alcoholism, Clinical and Experimental Research, 26*, 15S–19S.

Kamataki, T., Nunoya, K., Sakai, Y., Kushida, H., & Fujita, K. (1999). Genetic polymorphism of CYP2A6 in relation to cancer. *Mutation Research, 428*, 125–130.

Kelada, S. N., Kardia, S. L., Walker, A. H., Wein, A. J., Malkowicz, S. B., & Rebbeck, T. R. (2000). The glutathione S-transferase-mu and -theta genotypes in the etiology of prostate cancer: Genotype–environment interactions with smoking. *Cancer Epidemiology, Biomarkers & Prevention, 9*, 1329–1334.

Kharitonov, S. A., & Barnes, P. J. (2001). Exhaled markers of pulmonary disease. *American Journal of Respiratory and Critical Care Medicine, 163*, 1693–1722.

Kinney, P., Chillrud, S., Ramstrom, S., Ross, J., & Stansfeld, S. A. (2002). Exposure to multiple air toxics in New York city. *Environmental Health Perspectives, 110*(Suppl. 4), 539–546.

Kramer, M. S., Goulet, L., Lydon, J., Seguin, L., McNamara, H., Dassa, C., et al. (2001). Socio-economic disparities in preterm birth: Causal pathways and mechanisms. *Paediatric and Perinatal Epidemiology, 15*(Suppl. 2), 104–123.

Kyle, A. D., Woodruff, T. J., Buffler, P. A., & Davis, D. L. (2002). Use of an index to reflect the aggregate burden of long-term exposure to criteria air pollutants in the United States. *Environmental Health Perspectives, 110*(Suppl. 1), 95–102.

LaLonde, M. (1981). *A new perspective on the health of Canadians*. Government of Canada.

LaVeist, T. A. (2002). *Race, Ethnicity and Health*. San Francisco: Jose-Bass.

LaVeist, T. A., & Wallace, J. M., Jr. (2000). Health risk and inequitable distribution of liquor stores in African American neighborhood. *Social Science & Medicine, 51*, 613–617.

Lewis, S. J., Cherry, N. M., Niven, R. M., Barber, P. V., & Povey, A. C. (2002). GSTM1, GSTT1 and GSTP1 polymorphisms and lung cancer risk. *Cancer Letters, 180*, 165–171.

Luepker, R. V., Murray, D. M., Jacobs, D. R., Jr., Mittelmark, M. B., Bracht, N., Carlaw, R., et al. (1994). Community education for cardiovascular disease prevention: Risk factor changes in the Minnesota Heart Health Program. *American Journal of Public Health, 84*, 1383–1393.

Macintyre, S. (1997). The Black report and beyond: What are the issues? *Social Science & Medicine, 44*, 723–745.

Macintyre, S., Ellaway, A., & Cummins, S. (2002). Place effects on health: How can we conceptualise, operationalise and measure them? *Social Science & Medicine, 55*, 125–139.

Mauderly, J. (1993). Toxicological approaches to complex mixtures. *Environmental Health Perspectives, 101*, 155–165.

Medelsohn, J., Howley, P. M., Isreal, M. A., & Liotta, L. A. (2001). *The molecular basis of cancer* (2nd ed.). Philadelphia: WB Saunders.

Meyer, J. M., & Breitner, J. C. (1998). Multiple threshold model for the onset of Alzheimer's disease in the NAS-NRC twin panel. *American Journal of Medical Genetics, 81*, 92–97.

Meyer, J. M., & Ginsburg, G. S. (2002). The path to personalized medicine. *Current Opinion in Chemical Biology, 6*, 434–438.

Miller, D. P., Liu, G., De, V. I., Lynch, T. J., Wain, J. C., Su, L., et al. (2002). Combinations of the variant genotypes of GSTP1, GSTM1, and p53 are associated with an increased lung cancer risk. *Cancer Research, 62*, 2819–2823.

Minamoto, T., Mai, M., & Ronai, Z. (1999). Environmental factors as regulators and effectors of multistep carcinogenesis. *Carcinogenesis, 20*, 519–527.

Montuschi, P., Collins, J. V., Ciabattoni, G., Lazzeri, N., Corradi, M., Kharitonov, S. A., et al. (2000). Exhaled 8-isoprostane as an in vivo biomarker of lung oxidative stress in patients with COPD and healthy smokers. *American Journal of Respiratory and Critical Care Medicine, 162*, 1175–1177.

Morello-Frosch, R., Pastor, M., Porras, C., & Sadd, J. (2002). Environmental justice and regional inequality in southern California: Implications for future research. *Environmental Health Perspectives, 110*(Suppl. 2), 149–154.

Morland, K., Wing, S., & Diez, R. A. (2002). The contextual effect of the local food environment on residents' diets: The atherosclerosis risk in communities study. *American Journal of Public Health, 92*, 1761–1767.

Mucci, L. A., Wedren, S., Tamimi, R. M., Trichopoulos, D., & Adami, H. O. (2001). The role of gene–environment interaction in the aetiology of human cancer: Examples from cancers of the large bowel, lung and breast. *Journal of Internal Medicine, 249*, 477–493.

Murray, L. R. (2003). Sick and tired of being sick and tired: Scientific evidence, methods, and research implications for racial and ethnic disparities in occupational health. *American Journal of Public Health, 93*, 221–226.

Olsen, L. F., & Schaffer, W. M. (1990). Chaos versus noisy periodicity: Alternative hypotheses for childhood epidemics. *Science, 249*, 499–504.

Pargament, K. I., Maton, K. I., & Hess, R. E. (1992). *Religion and prevention in mental health.* Binghamton, NY: Hawthorne Press.

Pastorino, U., Berrino, F., Gervasio, A., Pesenti, V., Riboli, E., & Crosignani, P. (1984). Proportion of lung cancers due to occupational exposure. *International Journal of Cancer, 33*, 231–237.

Phillips, T. J., & Belknap, J. K. (2002). Complex-trait genetics: Emergence of multivariate strategies. *Nature Reviews. Neuroscience, 3*, 478–485.

Pitot, H. C. (2002a). *Fundamentals of oncology* (4th ed.). New York: Marcel Dekker, Inc.

Pitot, H. C. (2002b). The host–tumor relationship. In H. C. Pitot (Ed.), *Fundamentals of oncology* (4th ed., pp. 743–781). New York: Marcel Dekker, Inc.

Pope, C., Burnett, R., Thun, M., Calle, E., Krewski, D., Ito, K., et al. (2002). Lung cancer, cardiopulmonary mortality, and long-term exposure to fine particulate air pollution. *JAMA: The Journal of the American Medical Association, 287*, 1141.

Samet, J. M. (1995). What can we expect from epidemiologic studies of chemical mixtures? *Toxicology, 105*, 307–314.

Schuller, H. M. (2002). Mechanisms of smoking-related lung and pancreatic adenocarcinoma development. *Nature Reviews. Cancer, 2*, 455–463.

Sharma, A. M. (1998). The thrifty-genotype hypothesis and its implications for the study of complex genetic disorders in man. *Journal of Molecular Medicine, 76*, 568–571.

Shields, P. G. (1999). Molecular epidemiology of lung cancer. *Annals of Oncology, 10*(Suppl. 5), S7–S11.

Slattery, M. L., Curtin, K., Ma, K., Edwards, S., Schaffer, D., Anderson, K., et al. (2002). Diet activity and lifestyle associations with p53 mutations in colon tumors. *Cancer Epidemiology, Biomarkers & Prevention, 11*, 541–548.

Song, N., Tan, W., Xing, D., & Lin, D. (2001). CYP 1A1 polymorphism and risk of lung cancer in relation to tobacco smoking: A case–control study in China. *Carcinogenesis, 22*, 11–16.

Sorenson, M., Autrup, H., Hertel, O., Wallin, H., Knudson, E., & Logan, R. A. (2003). Personal exposure to PM2.5 and biomarkers of DNA damage. *Cancer Epidemiology, Biomarkers & Prevention, 12*, 191h–196h.

Stucker, I., Hirvonen, A., de, W. I., Cabelguenne, A., Mitrunen, K., Cenee, S., et al. (2002). Genetic polymorphisms of glutathione S-transferases as modulators of lung cancer susceptibility. *Carcinogenesis, 23*, 1475–1481.

Sunaga, N., Kohno, T., Yanagitani, N., Sugimura, H., Kunitoh, H., Tamura, T., et al. (2002). Contribution of the NQO1 and GSTT1 polymorphisms to lung adenocarcinoma susceptibility. *Cancer Epidemiology, Biomarkers & Prevention, 11*, 730–738.

Terry, L. (1964). *Smoking and health: A report of the Surgeon General.* Washington, DC: DHHS.

Tidd, C. W., Olsen, L. F., & Schaffer, W. M. (1993). The case for chaos in childhood epidemics. II. Predicting historical epidemics from mathematical models. *Proceedings. Biological Sciences, 254*, 257–273.

Ulrich, C. M., Kampman, E., Bigler, J., Schwartz, S. M., Chen, C., Bostick, R., et al. (1999). Colorectal adenomas and the C677T MTHFR polymorphism: Evidence for gene–environment interaction? *Cancer Epidemiology, Biomarkers & Prevention, 8*, 659–668.

Wadsworth, M. E. (1997). Health inequalities in the life course perspective. *Social Science & Medicine, 44*, 859–869.

Weisburger, J. H., & Chung, F. L. (2002). Mechanisms of chronic disease causation by nutritional factors and tobacco products and their prevention by tea polyphenols. *Food and Chemical Toxicology, 40*, 1145–1154.

Weiss, J. N., Garfinkel, A., Spano, M. L., & Ditto, W. L. (1994). Chaos and chaos control in biology. *The Journal of Clinical Investigation, 93*, 1355–1360.

Williams, D. R. (1999). Race, socioeconomic status, and health. The added effects of racism and discrimination. *Annals of the New York Academy of Sciences, 896*, 173–188.

Wilson, S., Jones, L., Coussens, C., & Hanna, K. (2002). *Cancer and the environment; Gene–environment interaction*. Washington, DC: The National Academy Press.

Yang, C. S., Chhabra, S. K., Hong, J. Y., & Smith, T. J. (2001). Mechanisms of inhibition of chemical toxicity and carcinogenesis by diallyl sulfide (DAS) and related compounds from garlic. *The Journal of Nutrition, 131*, 1041S–1045S.

Zang, E. A., & Wynder, E. L. (1998). Smoking trends in the United States between 1969 and 1995 based on patients hospitalized with non-smoking-related diseases. *Preventive Medicine, 27*, 854–861.

Zhao, B., Seow, A., Lee, E. J., Poh, W. T., Teh, M., Eng, P., et al. (2001). Dietary isothiocyanates, glutathione S-transferase -M1, -T1 polymorphisms and lung cancer risk among Chinese women in Singapore. *Cancer Epidemiology, Biomarkers & Prevention, 10*, 1063–1067.

Zmirou, D., Masclet, P., Boudet, C., Dor, F., & Dechenaux, J. (2000). Personal exposure to atmospheric polycyclic aromatic hydrocarbons in a general adult population and lung cancer risk assessment. *Journal of Occupational and Environmental Medicine, 42*, 121–126.

Zochbauer-Muller, S., Gazdar, A. F., & Minna, J. D. (2002). Molecular pathogenesis of lung cancer. *Annual Review of Physiology, 64*, 681–708.

13
Health Information Technology Policy Perspectives and Healthcare Disparities

Ruth Perot and Michael Christopher Gibbons

Brief Historical Overview of HIT Policy

Over the past few years, the federal government and the private sector have made progress toward the goal of enhancing healthcare delivery through improved use of health information technology (HIT) (Thompson & Brailer, 2004). This work began in 1998 when the National Committee on Vital and Health Statistics (NCVHS) in a paper entitled "Assuring a Health Dimension for the National Information Infrastructure" reported that the nation's information infrastructure could be an essential tool for promoting the nation's health (Thompson & Brailer). Since then, several other initiatives have helped to define the US approach to apply information and communication technologies to the health sector.

Four years later, in 2002, the Markle Foundation established the Connecting for Health Initiative, which brought together public and private leaders to discuss how to improve patient care by promoting standards for electronic medical information. The mission of this group was to identify and remove barriers to the growth of electronic connectivity in health care (Connecting for Health Collaborative, 2004). In March 2003, the Consolidated Health Informatics initiative involving HHS, the Departments of Defense, and Veterans Affairs, announced uniform standards for the electronic exchange of clinical health information that would be adopted across federal healthcare agencies. At the end of 2003, President Bush signed into law the Medicare Prescription Drug Improvement and Modernization Act of 2003. Among other things, this law required the Centers for Medicare and Medicaid Services to develop standards for electronic prescribing for use in electronic health records. It also called for the establishment of a new commission to develop guidance for interoperability standards (Thompson & Brailer, 2004).

In April of the next year, President Bush unveiled his "Technology and Innovation" agenda in which he announced a series of specific measures designed to inspire a new generation of American innovation. These included policies to encourage clean energy, assure better delivery of health care through technology, and expand access to high-speed Internet in every part of America (Bush, 2004). That same month, President Bush issued Executive Order 13335 calling for widespread adoption of interoperable Electronic Health Records within 10 years and established the position of National Coordinator for Health Information Technology. The Executive Order directed the National Coordinator to produce a report, within 90 days of operation, on the development and implementation of a strategic plan to guide the nationwide implementation of interoperable HIT in both the public and private sectors (Thompson & Brailer, 2004).

This executive order was largely based on several potential benefits of adopting HIT for the nation's healthcare system, providers, and consumers. The benefits to the healthcare consumer include (1) higher quality care, (2) reduction in medical errors, (3) fewer duplicate treatments and tests, (4) decrease in paperwork, (5) lower healthcare costs, (6) constant access to health information, and (7) expansion of access to affordable care. There were also several perceived benefits to public health. These include (1) early detection of infectious disease outbreaks around the country, (2) improved tracking of chronic disease management, (3) ability to gather deidentified data for research purposes, and (4) evaluation of health care based on value, enabled by the collection of price and quality information that can be compared (US DHHS, 2007).

In summer 2004, Connecting for Health released a "Preliminary Roadmap for Achieving Electronic Connectivity in Healthcare." This report suggested that the US should create a technical framework for connectivity. This network of networks as they called it would be built on the infrastructure of the Internet that would have safeguards to ensure privacy and security of all health information (Connecting for Health Collaborative, 2004). The roadmap also suggested the need for developing incentives to promote improvements in healthcare quality, and engaging the American public to develop and disseminate both general messages and messages tailored to specific audiences that will encourage greater citizen participation in health care through the use of technology. A central premise articulated in this document was that each patient would retain control and have direct access to all their health information as would any physician participating in the care of the patient (Connecting for Health Collaborative; Thompson & Brailer, 2004).

In 2005, the secretary of Health and Human Services established the American Health Information Community (AHIC). This group would function as a federal advisory body and would be composed of public and private sector individuals who represent a broad spectrum of healthcare stakeholders. The AHIC was established to make recommendations to the secretary on how to accelerate adoption of interoperable electronic health IT in a smooth, market-led way (US DHHS, 2007). In addition, the Office of the National Coordinator for Health Information Technology (ONC) was established within the Office of the Secretary at HHS.

In May 2006, the AHIC issued recommendations to the secretary of health regarding the utilization and standardization of electronic health records, secure patient–provider email messaging, and biosurveillance. In August, they provided recommendations on "Interoperability Specifications" that would enable the hundreds of different computer and data systems across the country to communicate effectively (Thompson & Brailer, 2004).

Finally, in August 2006, President Bush issued another Executive Order requiring all federal departments and agencies that purchase and deliver health care to use health IT that is based on interoperability standards recognized by the Secretary of HHS and proposed by AHIC. The Certification Commission for Healthcare Information Technology (CCHIT) certified the first 37 electronic health record products. These products met federal standards for minimum functionality, security, and interoperability (US DHHS, 2007).

In terms of congressional legislative activity, as of the 109th congressional session, US House and Senate legislators were considering approximately 41 pieces of legislation relating in some way to the role of technology in health care. Of these, only one, the Patient Safety and Quality Improvement Act of 2005, was signed into law (PL 109-41 signed on 7/29/05) (Healthcare Information and Management Systems Society, 2006). This bill promotes the adoption of national health information data sharing and HIT interoperability standards (Healthcare Information and Management Systems Society).

HIT Policy and Healthcare Disparities

As can be seen by the outline above, most of the national and federal policy work to date concerning HIT in health care has been in reference to issues related primarily to patient and provider utilization of Electronic Health Records. As it relates health-care disparities specifically, several policy gaps and opportunities are evident.

It is difficult to estimate how many providers currently use HIT in their practices. Thus, it is a challenge to understand if the nation's poor, minority, and otherwise disadvantaged populations are benefiting from the potential electronic health records in clinical care. The most reliable estimates to date suggest that only 9% of providers report using high-quality EHRs. This proportion rises to just 23.9% if providers using any type of EHR are included (Jha et al., 2006). More importantly, no nationally representative data are available; therefore, reliable national estimates are not possible regarding EHR adoption among safety net providers. In a study of Community Health Centers in California, less than 10% of centers were using elec-tronic systems to support individual patient care (Jha et al.). Based on this data, it appears that much work is still needed among all providers, but particularly among safety net providers who tend to lag behind in the adoption of new health technologies and medical innovations.

As has been discussed in the chapter on digital disparities, significant evidence exists in documenting differential access to and utilization of technology and the Internet among the nation's disadvantaged populations (see Chap. 8). These digital disparities are complex, nuanced, and multifaceted. The underlying causes of these disparities cannot be fully explained by socioeconomic and geographic factors. Indeed the nature and magnitude of these digital disparities will likely change. Some may diminish in magnitude or relevance while others may increase. Other disparities may also arise that are not currently recognized. As information technology plays an ever-increasing role in Americans' economic and social lives, the prospect that some people may not be able to take advantage of HIT innovations in health care may have significant implications for our nation's healthcare system (US Department of Commerce, 1999) and limit national efforts to reduce healthcare disparities.

Another policy opportunity with regard to healthcare disparities relates to patient adoption of EHRs. Whether or not the poor or minorities (or the general public) will buy into the notion of EHRs or other computer-based health technologies is still largely unknown. It appears that for the most part, the government, private sector businesses, and developers may largely be hoping that high-quality advertising, existing health needs, or the provision of high-quality health information will itself create significant demand for utilization of these products. While there may be some truth to this idea, in regard to improving healthcare disparities, operating under this assumption may, in terms of return on investment, prove faulty in a best case scenario or catastrophic in a worst case scenario (Gibbons, 2006).

Behavioral scientists have shown that while the provision of high-quality health information is a requisite for informed decision-making, information alone is insufficient to motivate significant behavior change in many patients, particularly over the long term (Carleton, Lasater, Assaf, Feldman, & McKinlay, 1995; Farquhar et al., 1990; *Health education and health behavior: Theory, research and practice*, 1997; Luepker et al., 1994). For example, consider the case of healthcare disparities among African-Americans with hypertension. Increasingly, various sociocultural factors, including culturally oriented diets and body appearance norms, are being recognized as being contributors to the problems of observed healthcare disparities in hypertension and cardiovascular diseases (Watkins, 2004).

It has been shown that among African-Americans, there is a belief that health outcomes may be ordained by God and therefore cannot be changed. This cultural belief among African-Americans has been called fatalism by medical researchers (Kressin & Petersen, 2001). It has been noted that this belief as well as other culturally determined attitudes and beliefs (myths) may impact decision-making among African-American patients and contribute to hypertensive disparities (Ferguson et al., 1998).

Additionally, some African-American men incorrectly described being healthy as being symptom-free and as a result, self-adjusted their hypertension medication usage depending on the existence of "symptoms." In addition, these men consider buying antihypertensive medications a luxury because of their high cost. They also think that seeking help for hypertension is a sign of weakness or laziness (Rose, Kim, Dennison, & Hill, 2000). These attitudes and beliefs may, in part, also be responsible for the existence of suboptimal medication adherence and inadequate self-monitoring of blood pressure among African-Americans (Chobanian et al., 2003). Although the evidence indicates that as many as 50% of all newly diagnosed hypertensive discontinue use of prescribed medications within 1 year and up to 50% of all remaining patients do not take their medications as prescribed (Friday, 1999), issues of poor medication adherence and inadequate self-monitoring of blood pressure are problems especially problematic among African-American patients (Artinian, Washington, & Templin, 2001; Friday; Hill et al., 1999; Rose et al.). In another example, some African-American men believe that seeking help for an illness or disease is a sign of weakness or laziness. It is possible that this belief may hinder the acceptance of EHRs and other technology-based health applications designed to enhance health care among this population. Obviously then, mistrust, misperceptions, and myths may impede medication compliance among African-American patients. To address these problems, additional research and targeted HIT disparities reduction policy initiatives will likely be needed.

While most of the federal policy work has targeted adoption of EHRs by providers, earlier chapters in this book provide the evidence to suggest that with respect to enhancing health care and reducing healthcare disparities, many other benefits potentially exist with the utilization of other new and emerging electronic technologies (Internet, smart medical devices, etc.). These products may do more than facilitate information transfer of medical information between providers and patients (Gibbons, 2005) (also see Chap. 14). While the current state of research on healthcare disparities and HIT does not permit precise quantification of this benefit, based on conservative estimates, it could be substantial. However, before this benefit can be realized, much more research needs to be done to enhance our understanding of the role culturally determined norms and behavioral factors may play in (1) the adoption of technology in the healthcare setting, (2) the utilization of technology, and (3) the potential impact of technology on minority and disadvantaged individuals' perceptions of the patient–provider relationship and trust in the healthcare system.

Finally, poor patient health literacy or limited English proficiency may limit a patient's ability to utilize emerging health technologies. Health literacy is defined as the ability to read and comprehend health-related materials (Baker, 1999). Approximately 40 million Americans, fully 25% of the US population, and 80% of English- and Spanish-speaking patients over the age of 60 suffer from inadequate literacy (Gazmararian et al., 1999; Weiss & Coyne, 1997). Low literacy rates are also prevalent among the poor, urban, and minority populations (Williams et al., 1995). Studies of low literate patients suggest that they are less likely to understand hospital discharge instructions or know essential information about diseases (Baker).

As among other minority and disadvantaged groups, many Latinos are less likely than others to use technologies such as computers and the Internet. In particular, those with less education, those with lower household incomes, and those who are over the age of 60 are least likely to be connected (Fox & Livingston, 2007). Overall, 29% of Hispanic adults have home broadband connections, compared with 43% of White adults.

As can be seen from the above discussion, several factors including HIT adoption rates among safety net providers, sociocultural beliefs and mistrust, literacy and English proficiency, and access to technology all mitigate against HIT adoption among disadvantaged populations. These factors also contribute to the existence of healthcare disparities (Smedley, Stith, & Nelson, 2003). Ignoring these issues when crafting HIT policy could ultimately impact the adoption, utilization, and business model for HIT investment nationally, limit the efficacy of healthcare improvements, and potentially increase healthcare disparities among these traditionally underserved and less connected populations of individuals.

HIT Healthcare Policy Recommendations and Principles

Given the above discussion, several opportunities for policy leadership in the area of HIT policy become evident. To move forward, policy initiatives should be built on the following *policy principles*:

1. The federal government has an essential leadership role to play in ensuring that communities of color and other underserved populations participate fully in HIT initiatives.
2. A key requisite to successful widespread adoption of HIT by patients from underserved communities is that *consumers* own personal health data and that privacy/confidentiality safeguards are essential and under their control. Accordingly, the federal government must increase its efforts to ensure privacy and security of personal health information in consultation with consumer representatives from diverse populations in the nation.
3. The goal of ensuring that most Americans have access to EHRs by 2014 cannot likely be reached unless there is a commitment to achieve universal broadband access to the Internet. Universal and affordable availability will be instrumental in attaining health parity, and anything less will likely lead to perpetuation and may exacerbate healthcare disparities.
4. Community partnerships are essential to facilitate trust and attain HIT adoption among underserved populations. Representatives from these communities need to be credibly involved in the development of policies, the conduct of HIT demonstrations, and the process of full-scale program implementation, research, and evaluation to help ensure success.
5. In terms of healthcare disparity reduction, HIT policy should be informed by the behavioral and communication as well as the clinical sciences and thereby be evidence based. Well meaning, but uniformed policymaking carries the potential of yielding minimal impact on healthcare disparities reduction and in some cases may exacerbate observed differences.

On the basis of the above policy principles, the following *policy recommendations* are made:

1. Fully fund current federal initiatives to provide critical resources to complete the goal of the President's Health Information Technology Executive Order such that most Americans will have an electronic health record by 2014, and ensure the inclusion of racial/ethnic and other underserved communities in such initiatives, which should also include informing clinical practice, interconnecting providers, personalizing care, and improving population health.
2. Establish public/private partnerships through which incentives, as well as technical and financial resources, can be directed to providers and consumers in minority and other underserved communities to help close the "digital divide."
3. Enact comprehensive legislation that will address the impact of HIT on healthcare disparities, to include

- Grants and other incentives to establish Healthcare Information Technology Empowerment Zones that demonstrate effective practices for promoting the adoption of HIT by consumers from vulnerable populations, as well as by providers who care for patients who are medically underserved and are impacted by health and/or digital disparities.
- Grants and contracts to assess the potential impact of nonadoption of HIT among providers serving racial/ethnic, low-income, and other vulnerable, medically underserved populations with respect to the possible exacerbation of health gaps in healthcare quality, treatment, and outcomes. Special efforts should be made to engage minority institutions and organizations in these efforts.
- Resources to support outreach efforts to promote HIT adoption by informing racial/ethnic and other underserved communities regarding HIT utilization options, benefits, and privacy safeguards. These initiatives should utilize activities and strategies that are culturally and linguistically appropriate and engage community stakeholders in the development, execution, and evaluation of such efforts.
- Policies to promote use of HIT in federally-funded programs, with the provision that targeted resources will be made available to healthcare providers in racial/ethnic and other underserved communities so that they will not be disadvantaged by such policies.

4. Formalize a relationship between the American Health Information Community and the National Institutes of Health (NIH), specifically the Office of Behavioral and Social Sciences Research (OBSSR) in the Office of the Director of the NIH and the National Center for Minority Health and Health Disparities (NCMHHD) at the NIH. This relationship should provide for permanent membership in one or more of the American Health Information Community workgroups by one or more representatives of the OBSSR and the NCMHHD. This will help to ensure that the AHIC remains informed of the latest evidence in regard to healthcare disparities as it relates to health information technologies. It will also serve to better link science with policy and position AHIC members/workgroups to make evidence-based recommendations to the secretary of HHS.

5. Establish a crosscutting Healthcare Disparities workgroup at the American Health Information Community. While it is conceivable that issues related to those of healthcare disparities reduction could arise within the context of one or more of the existing seven workgroups, given the current challenging scope of activities with these workgroups are charged, it is likely that difficulties in completing current tasks would arise if one or more of these groups attempted to deliberate the issues with regard to HIT and healthcare disparities to the same degree as their current topics of discussion. Rather, it would be advantageous to establish a workgroup charged to specifically consider such issues and to inform the secretary of the potential implications of the recommendations of the other seven workgroups and provide the secretary with a focused set of recommendations to address identified concerns, within the mandate of the American Health Information Community.

Despite the technological challenges that threaten to impede attaining a technology-enhanced healthcare system, several exciting policy opportunities exist, and much progress has been made. With continued hard work and dedicated policy leadership, success is entirely achievable.

References

Artinian, N. T., Washington, O. G., & Templin, T. N. (2001). Effects of home telemonitoring and community-based monitoring on blood pressure control in urban African Americans: A pilot study. *Heart Lung, 30*, 191–199.

Baker, D. W. (1999). Reading between the lines: Deciphering the connections between literacy and health. *Journal of General Internal Medicine, 14*, 315–317.

Bush, G. W. (2004). *A new generation of American innovation.* http://www.whitehouse.gov/infocus/technology/economic_policy200404/chap1.html [On-line].

Carleton, R. A., Lasater, T. M., Assaf, A. R., Feldman, H. A., & McKinlay, S. (1995). The Pawtucket Heart Health Program: Community changes in cardiovascular risk factors and projected disease risk. *American Journal of Public Health, 85*, 777–785.

Chobanian, A. V., Bakris, G. L., Black, H. R., Cushman, W. C., Green, L. A., Izzo, J. L., Jr., et al. (2003). The seventh report of the Joint National Committee on prevention, detection, evaluation, and treatment of high blood pressure: The JNC 7 report. *JAMA: The Journal of the American Medical Association, 289*, 2560–2572.

Connecting For Health Collaborative. (2004). *Achieving electronic connectivity in healthcare; A preliminary roadmap from the nation's public and private sector healthcare leaders.* Washington, DC: The Markle Foundation.

Farquhar, J. W., Fortmann, S. P., Flora, J. A., Taylor, C. B., Haskell, W. L., Williams, P. T., et al. (1990). Effects of communitywide education on cardiovascular disease risk factors. The Stanford Five-City Project. *JAMA: The Journal of the American Medical Association, 264*, 359–365.

Ferguson, J. A., Weinberger, M., Westmoreland, G. R., Mamlin, L. A., Segar, D. S., Greene, J. Y., et al. (1998). Racial disparity in cardiac decision making: Results from patient focus groups. *Archives of Internal Medicine, 158*, 1450–1453.

Fox, S., & Livingston, G. (2007). *Latinos online.* Washington, DC: Pew Charitable Trusts.

Friday, G. H. (1999). Antihypertensive medication compliance in African-American stroke patients: Behavioral epidemiology and interventions. *Neuroepidemiology, 18*, 223–230.

Gazmararian, J. A., Baker, D. W., Williams, M. V., Parker, R. M., Scott, T. L., Green, D. C., et al. (1999). Health literacy among Medicare enrollees in a managed care organization. *JAMA: The Journal of the American Medical Association, 281*, 545–551.

Gibbons, M. C. (2005). A historical overview of health disparities and the potential of eHealth solutions. *Journal of Medical Internet Research, 7*, e50.

Gibbons, M. C. (2006). Health inequalities and emerging themes in compunetics. *Studies in Health Technology and Informatics, 121*, 62–69.

Health education and health behavior: Theory, research and practice (2nd ed.). (1997). San Fransisco: Jose-Bass.

Healthcare Information and Management Systems Society. (2006). *Health IT legislative crosswalk.* Washington, DC: Healthcare Information and Management Systems Society.

Hill, M., Bone, L., Kim, M., Miller, D., Dennison, C., & Levine, D. (1999). Barriers to hypertension care and control in young urban black men. *American Journal of Hypertension, 12*, 951–958.

Jha, A. K., Ferris, T. G., Donelan, K., DesRoches, C., Shields, A., Rosenbaum, S., et al. (2006). How common are electronic health records in the United States? A summary of the evidence. *Health Affairs (Project Hope), 25*, w496–w507.

Kressin, N. R., & Petersen, L. A. (2001). Racial differences in the use of invasive cardiovascular procedures: Review of the literature and prescription for future research. *Annals of Internal Medicine, 135*, 352–366.

Luepker, R. V., Murray, D. M., Jacobs, D. R., Jr., Mittelmark, M. B., Bracht, N., Carlaw, R., et al. (1994). Community education for cardiovascular disease prevention: Risk factor changes in the Minnesota Heart Health Program. *American Journal of Public Health, 84*, 1383–1393.

Rose, L., Kim, M., Dennison, C., & Hill, M. (2000). The context of adherence for African-Americans with high blood pressure. *Journal of Advanced Nursing, 32*, 587–594.

Smedley, B. D., Stith, A. Y., & Nelson, A. R. (2003). *Unequal treatment: Confronting racial and ethnic disparities in healthcare.* Washington, DC: The National Academy Press.

Thompson, T., & Brailer, D. (2004). *The decade of health information technology: Delivering consumer-centric and information-rich health care – Framework for strategic action.* Department of Health and Human Services [On-line]. Available: www.hhs.gov.healthit

US Department of Commerce, N. T. a. I. A. (1999). *The digital divide summit.* http://www.ntia.doc.gov/ntiahome/digitaldivide/summit/[On-line].

US DHHS. (2007). *Health information technology initiative major accomplishments: 2004–2006.* Washington, DC: Government Printing Office.

Watkins, L. O. (2004). Perspectives on coronary heart disease in African Americans. *Reviews in Cardiovascular Medicine, 5*(Suppl. 3), S3–S13.

Weiss, B. D., & Coyne, C. (1997). Communicating with patients who cannot read. *The New England Journal of Medicine, 337*, 272–274.

Williams, M. V., Parker, R. M., Baker, D. W., Parikh, N. S., Pitkin, K., Coates, W. C., et al. (1995). Inadequate functional health literacy among patients at two public hospitals. *JAMA: The Journal of the American Medical Association, 274*, 1677–1682.

14
Disparities and eHealth: Achieving the Promise and the Potential

Michael Christopher Gibbons

Healthcare Disparities

Over the last two decades, research from several distinct lines of investigation have coalesced to underscore the relationship between medical care, biophysiologic processes, and sociocultural and other environmental influences on healthcare outcomes generally and healthcare disparities specifically (see Chaps. 1–5). In the early 1980s, researchers examining variability in clinical practice patterns found nonrandom distributions in care across geographic locations. In the mid-1980s, the report of the Secretary's Task Forces on Black and Minority Health highlighted the fact that the health of Blacks and minorities significantly lagged behind that of Whites in the US (Department of Health and Human Services, 1985). By the early 1990s, large scale epidemiologic studies confirmed earlier findings of nonrandom distribution of clinical practice patterns and the association between substandard care with low income and minority patients. These early findings encouraged a focus on healthcare quality problems with the US healthcare system, which revealed that problems associated with quality and healthcare disparities were in fact linked and should be considered together. In the case of healthcare disparities, the more recent attempts to address disparities have in most cases yielded disappointing results. As such, efforts were undertaken to clarify better the impact of "nonmedical" communications and social factors on healthcare disparities and healthcare outcomes. These investigations highlighted the need to integrate better the biomedical and sociobehavioral disciplines in current health care and clinical practice to improve quality and address disparities among an increasingly diverse population. They also highlighted the fact that communication barriers, literacy, as well as cultural and behavioral influences likely play a far more significant role in healthcare disparities than previously appreciated by the broader medical community.

The Future of Health Care

Several factors impacting the nature and practice of health care itself are also suggesting the need for the healthcare system to improve its understanding and responsiveness to "nonmedical" communications and socioenvironmental factors. These include (1) the changing nature of health care in America, (2) the existence of healthcare disparities, and (3) the increasing pervasiveness of the Internet in American life.

In the US, over the last century, many acute and communicable diseases have either vanished or become much less prevalent. Over the same time period, there has been a rise in the prevalence of chronic conditions and diseases. Growing proportions of the population are living with chronic diseases. Approximately 60% of UK citizens and 50% of US citizens report having at least one chronic disease (IOM Committee on Quality of Healthcare in America, 2001; National Health Service, 2004). These numbers are expected to rise further in the near future. Fragmented healthcare delivery systems and significant proportions of individuals with multiple co-occurring disease conditions contribute directly to poor quality care, unnecessary medical errors, and poor patient outcomes (IOM Committee on Quality of Healthcare in America; National Health Service). Western healthcare systems are largely oriented toward acute episodic inpatient treatment and, as such, have only limited ability, in their current configurations to respond adequately to these growing concerns. A shift from acute, inpatient treatment to chronic, community-based, patient-centered, guided self-care and health risk management will demand an improved understanding of "nontraditional medical factors" that significantly impact patient adherence, compliance, satisfaction, and outcomes.

Effective chronic care, unlike acute treatment care, is a much more collaborative process between patients and providers. Much of this community-based care will be provided by nonphysician healthcare professionals, family members, friends, and associates (IOM Committee on Quality of Healthcare in America, 2001; National Health Service, 2004).

The Existence of Healthcare Disparities

While the existence of healthcare disparities can no longer be credibly disputed, there currently exists little consensus regarding the causes and especially the solutions for these disparities. Increasingly, however, scientists and policy makers agree that both the causes and solutions are likely to be complex, multifaceted, and interrelated. By definition, disparities are a group or population phenomenon. Individuals do not have disparities. Rather, disparities are racial or ethnic differences in the quality, outcomes, or access to health care that are not due to clinical needs, preferences, and appropriateness of medical interventions. Thus while disparities are measured at the population level, most healthcare interventions to date propose targeting individual patients and/or providers. While to some this may seem inappropriate, the truth is that both are needed because disparities can neither be comprehensively characterized nor understood by only considering population level data, nor can they be successfully reduced and eliminated by interventions only targeting individuals. Clearer characterizations of disparities will emerge when scientists are able to collectively analyze and integrate data from the cellular and molecular level with that from the individual or behavioral level in the context of community, neighborhood, and societal level data to understand the cause and development of healthcare disparities. Many traditional health care and health services research methodologies are inadequate to accomplish this task. Not only new analytic techniques and approaches are needed but also the power of computer technologies will be required to enable the collection, storage, and analysis of these increasingly large and diverse data sets. Novel computer-based visualization techniques will also be important to help turn this data into useable knowledge by health services planners and healthcare policy makers. Finally, increasingly sophisticated computer-based methodologies will be needed to protect the identity and privacy of users while enabling appropriate authentication of authorized parties to use available data. As we go forward, it becomes a challenge to conceptualize how disparities in health and health care might be adequately understood or addressed in the absence of novel and powerful computer technologies.

The Future of the Internet and Computer Technologies in Health Care

Since the early days of the Internet, the numbers of online health seekers have swelled to approximately 113 million people. During this time, significant shifts in the practices and habits of online health seekers were evident. These individuals increasingly became informed and empowered, which at times led to some friction with some healthcare providers. Over time, however, many providers themselves began using the Internet to enhance their medical knowledge and patient care services. The rapid growth in online health activities was fueled in part by significant increases in home broadband and wireless access which in turn enabled many health seekers to engage in much more intense health information seeking activities.

These online health seekers are drawn to the convenience and anonymity of online health information. They are generally able to find what they are looking for and report that the Internet is increasingly helping them to connect to emotional support and practical help for dealing with their health issues. The Internet also provides many online opportunities to provide support by helping other online health seekers keep up with the latest information and health news. As the Internet has matured, there has been an increasing interest in wellness activities and resources in addition to disease-oriented information.

In addition to the external pressures from newly empowered and increasingly connected e-patients, there is increasing internal interest in the role of technology in health care. Many have predicted a coming revolution in health care similar to the transformations that occurred in the finance and retail industries upon the widespread adoption of computer technology (Abrams, 2006; Crane & Raymond, 2003; Gibbons, 2005, 2006b). Indeed, health professionals today recognize that a significant portion of their activities involve the management of information. As such, information technology has become central to health communication, research, and practice (*Medical informatics*, 2001). To date, large drug databases may be searched in seconds for potential drug interactions, electrocardiograms are analyzed via computers, and patients' vital signs are constantly monitored in intensive care units and operating rooms by computers (*Medical Informatics*). Advanced decision support and telemedical tools, electronic health records, computerized physician order entry systems, remote monitoring, early detection, and advanced warning systems are being developed and promise to significantly impact medical care in a variety of ways (*Medical Informatics*). The fields of Medical Informatics, Bioinformatics, and eHealth have themselves all undergone rapid evolution and expansion over the past few years. These developments portend a future healthcare system where all of an individual's health information can be available to any patient or provider from any place at anytime. Once achieved, it may significantly reduce medical decision-making errors due to the lack of needed information. This in turn should improve the quality of health care and may lead to improvements in healthcare disparities.

To completely understand the true magnitude and potential of future information and communications technologies on the healthcare system and health outcomes, the role of the Internet (and the personal computer) must be put into perspective. Historically, the printing press was *the* biggest innovation in communications until the telegraph was developed. Although printing remained the key format for mass messages for years afterward, the telegraph, for the first time in history, allowed instant communication over long distances. Soon telegraph usage faded as the radio became easy to use. About the same time, the telephone became the fastest way to communicate person-to-person. But, as television content and quality improved, it (TV) became the dominant form of communication technology. Now the Internet has been developed. Newspapers, radio, telephones, and television are seemingly being rolled into this single information medium, whose pervasiveness and ease of use is largely unheralded (Anderson, 2005). As noted in the previous chapters, consumers are particularly drawn to the convenience, anonymity, and simplicity the Web offers when searching for health or medical information. These factors also appear to have been of primary importance in the rise and fall of past communications technologies. Today, many healthcare providers have also come to rely on the Internet as one source of medical information (Powell, Darvell, & Gray, 2003), while some have even suggested that search engines like Google may one day assist with diagnostic decision-making (Tang & Ng, 2006).

The development of this medium (the Internet & computer technologies), however, is not complete. As such, it is reasonable to conclude that the full potential of Internet & computer technologies has not been achieved. Along these lines, the potential of technology may extend well beyond that of facilitating global information transfer.

The term Web 2.0 is increasingly being used to describe the next generation of the Internet. Although currently Web 2.0 is not precisely defined, what seems clear is that Web 2.0 enthusiasts and applications are primarily concerned with the notion of going beyond using the Internet for information sharing to enabling dynamic, interactive, collaborative experiences that are increasingly embedded in the daily activities of people's lives (Giustini, 2006). Wikis, blogs/photoblogs, podcasts, vodcasts, and skype are the first iterations of these collaboration ware tools that rely on the Internet and carry the potential of complementing, improving, and adding new collaborative dimensions to the clinicomedical interventions and treatments (Boulos, Maramba, & Wheeler, 2006).

Even as this Web 2.0 evolution has scarcely begun, the next "revolution" in the Internet is in sight, enabled not by novel applications or online content, but by technological advances that are heralding the so-called ubiquitous computing and communication era (International Telecommunications Union, 2005). This idea of technological ubiquity suggests that the increasing "availability" of processing power will be accompanied by its decreasing "visibility." As such, "the most profound technologies will be those that disappear...they weave themselves into the fabric of everyday life until they are indistinguishable from it" (International Telecommunications Union). This is made possible, in part, by miniaturization and by embedding short-range mobile transceivers into a wide array of household and everyday items. This will then enable new forms of communication between people, between people and things, and between things themselves (International Telecommunications Union). A new dimension will be added to the world of information and communication that will not only enable information and communication anytime for anyone at any place, but also enable connectivity between things (International Telecommunications Union) and yield an entirely new dynamic network dubbed an Internet of Things. The Internet of Things is not science fiction nor industry hype, but is based on solid technological advances and visions of network ubiquity that are zealously being realized (International Telecommunications Union) through global research efforts and entrepreneurial innovation. The realization of an Internet of Things, which in turn is connected to the network of networks (the Internet), will depend on technical innovation in a number of important fields including wireless sensors and nanotechnology (International Telecommunications Union).

The major technological advances upon which this Internet of Things is predicated are (1) a reliable system of hardware/device identification. This will enable one device to be distinguishable from another on a network of devices (International Telecommunications Union, 2005). To connect everyday objects and devices to large databases, networks, and the Internet, a simple, unobtrusive, and cost-effective system of item identification is crucial. Only then can data about things be collected and processed. Radio-frequency identification (RFID) offers this functionality (International Telecommunications Union). RFID technology uses radio waves to identify items and is seen as one of the future pivotal enablers of the Internet (International Telecommunications Union). It can be thought of as the next generation of bar codes. RFID systems offer much more though in that they can track items in real-time to yield important information about their location and status (International Telecommunications Union). Early applications of RFID include automatic highway toll collection, pharmaceuticals (for the prevention of counterfeiting), and e-health (for patient monitoring). RFID tags are even being implanted under human skin for medical purposes and being embedded in mobile phones (International Telecommunications Union). (2) The ability to detect changes in the physical status of things is essential for recording changes in the local environment of the device. Here, sensor technology will enable things to detect changes in the local physical environment of the sensor. Sensors will collect data from their environment thus generating information and raising awareness about context (International Telecommunications Union). The combination of RFID, remote sensing technology, and wireless Internet can enable the seamless transport of physiologic or environmental data to providers and researchers in real time almost without notice to the patient. Likewise, providers will be able to respond and remotely instruct the devices themselves to do things in response to detected external information. (3) Finally, advances in nanotechnology and miniaturization, particularly of microprocessors, will enable the distribution of computer processing power to the edges of the network rather than in a central processing unit of a server or desktop computer. This suggests the possibility of things and devices at the edges of the network having the ability to detect change in the local environment, analyze the changes, and respond appropriately within preprogrammed parameters (International Telecommunications Union) *without* the need for additional human intervention to determine a response. "Smart things" as such devices have been called imply a certain processing power and reaction to external stimuli. Scientists are using their imagination to develop new devices and appliances such as intelligent ovens that can be controlled through phones or the Internet, online refrigerators, and networked blinds that respond automatically to the intensity of sunlight coming in through the windows. Ultimately, the Internet of Things will enable the realization of a vision of a fully interactive and responsive networked environment (International Telecommunications Union).

The Promise and the Potential in Healthcare Disparities

In the end, the potential impact of technology on health care and disparities should neither be overlooked nor underestimated. This impact will undoubtedly go far beyond mere information sharing between patients, providers, and healthcare systems, to enabling clinical research and experiential medicobehavioral interventions not currently conceivable. The potential benefits of technological advances on healthcare disparities are likely to be seen in at least three areas. The increased use of computer technologies in health care could enable enhanced characterizations of the causes and determinants of healthcare disparities. Emerging disciplines like Populomics (see Chap. 11) which rely on nontraditional transdisciplinary research models and methodologies like the Sociobiologic Integrative model (see Chap. 12) along with other methodologic advances may lead to characterizations of population level data to enable the development of "community (population) arrays" or community-wide risk profiles and permit the real-time integrative and simultaneous utilization of vast amounts of behavioral-, biological-, and community-level information to help us better understand the evolution of healthcare disparities (Gibbons, 2005).

Computer technologies in health care could also enable the design of novel and more effective clinical and behavioral healthcare interventions. By relying on user-centered design strategies in the development of future ehealth technologies (see Chap. 10), we may be able to turn sociocultural beliefs and behaviors, which may limit clinical efficacy, into tailored design features that facilitate the diffusion and adoption of powerful health tools including EMRs and other technologies in health care.

Computer technologies in health care may also enhance current interventions. For example, the use of Community Health Workers (CHWs) has been advocated by several groups, including the Institute of Medicine, as one culturally appropriate approach to help address healthcare disparities (Gibbons, 2006a, 2006b; Smedley, Stith, & Nelson, 2003). CHWs are individuals who are indigenous to the target community who work with both providers and community members to improve quality of health care, health status, and access to healthcare services provided to community members. Because they are from the target community, they are trusted by the community and are often more knowledgeable about community norms and culture than the outside "experts." Such individuals have been referred to by more than 30 different names, including navigators, lay health advisors, and health aides. Generally, however, the title Community Health Worker is most commonly used to describe these paraprofessionals (Rosenthal, 1998). In part, because of skyrocketing healthcare costs, health disparities, and worsening differentials in access to care, interest, and research is reemerging around the possible widespread utilization of CHWs (Gibbons, 2006a, 2006b; Nittoli & Giloth, 1997).

Evidence suggests that strategies integrating information technology with culturally appropriate behavioral interventions may have significant promise in improving access to care, enhancing the quality and satisfaction with care, and potentially reducing disparities. Additionally, many investigators agree that approaches and strategies that involve community members will be needed to adequately address disparities in health care. A CHW-mediated care delivery model has significant potential to promote health and reduce well-recognized disparities in underserved communities, including those in cardiovascular diseases (Capitman, Bhalotra, Calderon-Rosado, & Gibbons, 2003; Lewin et al., 2003; Nittoli & Giloth, 1997; Smedley et al., 2003).

While the CHW model holds significant promise, even the best trained and hardest working CHWs using paper and pencil along with word of mouth communication strategies can accomplish only a finite amount of work. The data and information they gather must be entered into an appropriate computer system, cleaned, verified, and then at some point after the data was initially obtained made available for use by providers for analysis or intervention. Consider, however, the possibilities of trained CHWs working in collaboration with healthcare providers. Consider the potential of having these workers networked to each other via laptop computers with wireless broad band connections to the Internet. Instantly, a wealth of patient education, medication, community health resources, and other healthcare information is available at the finger tips of the worker, at anytime or any place, to aid in the education, motivation, or compliance of any patient. Consider the additional possibilities if these laptops were connected directly to the providers overseeing the CHW activities. These providers could at any time, and in real time, conceivably know a virtually limitless amount of physiologic (blood pressure, heart rate, wound healing progress, etc.) data about a potentially infinite number of patients who are not hospitalized, not in a clinic or emergency room, and could even be homeless or relaxing in bed reading a book! If ten CHWs go into the field and each takes the blood pressure of ten individuals and transmit that information back to the hospital or clinic, the provider would then be able to instantly know the blood pressures of 100 people, in real time. He could then respond as appropriate, if needed. With the aid of a simple digital camera, any patient the CHW interacts with could potentially also interact with his or her provider without leaving trusted, familiar surroundings in their communities! This could potentially go a long way toward improving access to care for those who traditionally mistrust the healthcare system and are otherwise underserved or hard to reach!

These computer-based healthcare interventions will not likely be limited by contemporary barriers of geographic proximity to health care, literacy, language, or human error. In this future healthcare system, Human to Human (H2H) connectivity will enable providers and healthcare systems to stay in audio and visual contact as needed. Human to Thing (H2T) connectivity will enable both providers and patients to know about the health status of individuals or populations and their surroundings at any time, in real time, prior to the need for and after hospitalization. Thing to Thing (T2T) connectivity (the Internet of things) will mean the development of "intelligent devices" that can make decisions and do things independent of the "human element." Thus, the potential opportunity and impact of racial bias and discrimination in health care should be minimized. In this future healthcare system, clinicians and researchers can know and understand how social, environmental, and biological factors collectively contribute to ill health. Health risks can then be managed in the homes and communities of the patients *before* these health risks become diseases and *before* patients even need to go to the hospital. In this future healthcare system, clinical interventions are delivered via a variety of formats including the Web, game console, interactive TV, cell phone, and PDAs, not just in person. In this future healthcare system, even the efficacy of traditional personal interventions could also be enhanced via technological adjuncts to treatment or care. Here, "clinical" interventions can be delivered anywhere and at any time as needed by patients. Health technology will enable exquisite mass customization and tailoring to the unique needs of each patient in large populations. Finally, in this healthcare system of the future, health care is proactive, helping patients manage their health risks. It will no longer be just reactive, providing heroic medical interventions if you are able to get to a hospital. Patients will no longer delay seeking care because they will be receiving it all the time. Smart devices equipped with evidence-based algorithms will have the potential to drastically reduce the number of medical errors that are made, while health information would be always accessible to both provider and patients in the most understandable formats for each. Thus, over time, there exists real potential to make significant impact toward the goal of reducing and eliminating disparities in healthcare access, utilization, and outcomes.

Research Needs, Gaps, and Policy Opportunities

The vision for the technology-based improvements in healthcare disparities is not based on mere speculation. Each portion of this vision is the current subject of intense research. A vast and diverse array of clinical and bench scientists, engineers, informaticists and informaticians, populations and system scientists across the globe are avidly working to add to the scientific knowledge base and build their piece of the puzzle. The preceding chapters of this book have attempted to introduce the reader to some of the research and activities in these areas.

To achieve this vision, sustained leadership and effort in several areas will be needed. The inherent complexities underlying the causes of chronic disease and healthcare disparities suggest the need for science to go beyond the historical reductionistic approach to discovery and intervention. To achieve the vision, greater integration of knowledge across the biomolecular and population sciences will be necessary. To maintain an artificial separation between biologic and population sciences is to study health and disease without respect for the contexts in which people live. Disparities can neither be completely characterized nor understood without an in-depth appreciation of both socioenvironmental and biomolecular contributors. Such an integration of knowledge will lead to a better understanding of the biomolecular mechanisms through which sociobehavioral factors operate to influence health outcomes generally and healthcare disparities specifically.

Secondly, a broader vision for the role of technology in health care will be needed. The ultimate limits of this vision cannot, at this time, be clearly defined largely because the technologies upon which these advances will be based are themselves still developing and evolving. What is clear is that the potential value of these technologies will go far beyond surveillance systems, early detection and monitoring, and information sharing. As the telegraph, telephone, and television profoundly changed human existence in ways not conceivable by their inventors, we are living within the evolution of an Internet revolution which is having the same effect. The challenge before us is to find novel ways that this technology and the societal changes which it brings (e-patients, smart devices, Internet of things) can be harnessed for the betterment of clinical care, healthcare outcomes, and the reduction of healthcare disparities.

Consequent with the increasing empowerment of patients will be the need for a greater patient orientation in health care. Currently, western healthcare systems are designed to maximize the efficiencies and conveniences of providers and administrators. Significant variability in the quality of care, escalating costs and fragmented organizational structures, and financing systems exist in a system designed to ameliorate acute episodic illness. Collectively, these factors along with other behavioral, biologic, and sociocultural factors contribute to the existence and seeming intractability of healthcare disparities. Research evaluating novel patient-centered, home- and community-based, chronic disease and prevention-oriented healthcare delivery, and financing systems is needed.

Finally, sustained health care and disparities policy leadership will be needed. The financial and infrastructural barriers impeding technological advancements in health care and healthcare disparities may seem insurmountable. Leaders who recognize the potential of technology and can work collaboratively across party lines will be the ones best able to galvanize resources and sustain a national commitment to an ideal of the best healthcare system in the world ... for every citizen in America.

References

Abrams, D. B. (2006). Applying transdisciplinary research strategies to understanding and eliminating health disparities. *Health Education & Behavior, 33*, 515–531.

Anderson, J. (2005). *Imagining the internet: Personalities, predictions and perspectives.* Lanham, MD: Rowman & Littlefield Publishers, Inc.

Boulos, M. N., Maramba, I., & Wheeler, S. (2006). Wikis, blogs and podcasts: A new generation of Web-based tools for virtual collaborative clinical practice and education. *BMC Medical Education, 6*, 41.

Capitman, J., Bhalotra, S. M., Calderon-Rosado, V., & Gibbons, M. C. (2003). *Cancer prevention and treatment demonstration for racial and ethnic minorities: Evidence report and evidence-based recommendations (Rep. No. 500-00-0031).* US Department of Health and Human Services.

Crane, R., & Raymond, B. (2003). Fulfilling the potential of clinical information systems. *The Permanente Journal, 7*, 62–67.

Department of Health and Human Services. (1985). *REPORT OF THE SECRETARY'S TASK FORCES ON BLACK AND MINORITY HEALTH.* Washington, DC: DHHS.

Gibbons, M. C. (2005). A historical overview of health disparities and the potential of eHealth solutions. *Journal of Medical Internet Research, 7*, e50.

Gibbons, M. C. (2006a). Common ground: Exploring policy approaches to addressing racial disparities from the left and the right. *The Journal of Healthcare Law and Policy, 9*, 48–76.

Gibbons, M. C. (2006b). Health inequalities and emerging themes in compunetics. *Studies in Health Technology and Informatics, 121*, 62–69.

Giustini, D. (2006). How Web 2.0 is changing medicine. *British Medical Journal, 333*, 1283–1284.

International Telecommunications Union. (2005). *The Internet of things (Rep. No. 377-05).* Geneva, Switzerland: The International Telecommunication Union.

IOM Committee on Quality of Healthcare in America. (2001). *Crossing the quality chasm: A new health system for the 21st century.* Washington, DC: The National Academy Press.

Lewin, S. A., Dick, J., Zwarenstein, M., Aja, G., van Wyk, B., Bosch-Capblanch, X., et al. (2003). Lay health workers in primary and community health care (Rep. No. CD004015.pub2). *The Cochrane Database of Systematic Reviews.*

Medical informatics (2nd ed.). (2001). New York: Springer.

National Health Service. (2004). *Chronic disease management: A compendium of information.* London, England: UK Department of Health.

Nittoli, J. M., & Giloth, R. P. (1997). New careers revisited: Paraprofessional job creation for low-income communities. *Social Policy, Winter*, 44–61.

Powell, J. A., Darvell, M., & Gray, J. A. (2003). The doctor, the patient and the world-wide web: How the internet is changing healthcare. *Journal of the Royal Society of Medicine, 96*, 74–76.

Rosenthal, E. L. (1998). *The final report of the national community health advisor study* Baltimore: Annie E. Casey Foundation.

Smedley, B. D., Stith, A. Y., & Nelson, A. R. (2003). *Unequal treatment: Confronting racial and ethnic disparities in healthcare*. Washington, DC: The National Academy Press.

Tang, H., & Ng, J. H. (2006). Googling for a diagnosis – Use of Google as a diagnostic aid: Internet based study. *British Medical Journal, 333*, 1143–1145.

Author Index

Subject Index